TRAPPED WITHIN

TRAPPED WITHIN

A TRUE STORY ABOUT SURVIVAL, RECOVERY, LOVE, AND HOPE

JO ANN GLIM

Published by: Stemma Books LLC

PO Box 174, Bradenton, FL 34206

JoAnnGlim.author@gmail.com

www.JoAnnGlim.com

ISBN: 978-0-9888129-9-4 (Paperback)
ISBN: 978-0-9888129-8-7 (eBook)

LCN: TX

Category: Body, Mind, & Spirit / Family Relationships / Inspiration

Edited by Dot and Dash LLC: www.dotanddashllc.com

Cover Design / Formatting by 99Designs - C7 creativezone

Print Interior Design by Eden Graphics www.edengraphics.net

eBook Formatting by Day Agency: www.dayagency.com

Printed in the United States of America

DEDICATED TO:

My amazing husband,

Bill

BILL AND I so greatly appreciate the men and women who tenderly treat the sick and dying, and those in need of healing.

To all shadow angels—family, friends, and strangers—you are the touch of heaven who instinctively reach out to others when they need love and consoling the most.

Blessed are the caregivers with loving hearts. You are the unsung heroes and heroines who tend to the daily routines of life for yourself and the incapacitated with no thought of accolades.

You are all amazing. From one who needed you... a heartfelt thank you.

I hope you'll enjoy this book. If you do, please share your thoughts by leaving a review (five stars means you loved it). We appreciate you taking the time to tell others what you think. Word of mouth is vital to reach those who would benefit from this story. We gratefully appreciate your time. Thank you.

TABLE OF CONTENTS

PART SIX – Transitions to a New Normal

PART SEVEN – Lessons Learned

RESOURCES

PREFACE

THIS STORY IS WRITTEN to offer encouragement to stroke survivors, hope to their family members and caretakers, and understanding to medical professionals or anyone interested in knowing what it's like to be Trapped Within your own body.

When I wrote the first draft of this book, the fingers of my right hand did not have the strength to move properly. They rested on the keyboard so often and spit out so many strings of letters instead of words that the computer refused to spellcheck. To that I said, "Ooooooooooo Kkkkkkkkkkk, I'll find another way," and I did. I wrote a good deal of the first draft using only my left hand.

It's my hope that by sharing my personal story, it'll remove some of the mystery from this debilitating disease when told from a survivor's point of view.

FOREWORD

It has been my pleasure to know Jo Ann Glim since 1998, when she entered my speech-pathology office offering to be a volunteer in a new program that paired stroke survivors with persons whom had just sustained a stroke.

She had an ever-present smile and a spirit that lit up a room. She progressed through the learning process to become a volunteer and graduated with eagerness seen in adults who were embarking on an adventure.

She was always ready to visit with new stroke survivors and let them know that there was a life after "disaster." She was an inspiration to them, as well as to me.

I know that this book will touch the lives of even more people. I have enjoyed my friendship with Jo Ann and am honored to be able to write this foreword.

—Tami Spyker Goudy,
Supervisor, Stroke Support Peer Visitor Program

PROLOGUE

My MOTHER WAS FIFTY-ONE years and seven months when she endured a stroke. She died three days later. I was with her throughout the ordeal. I was fourteen years old.

That experience molded me into the person I am today. I eat sensibly and exercise regularly. In fact, I enjoy healthy food and being physically active. I don't smoke, don't drink—never did. I don't preach to anyone who has chosen living in a way other than my own. This is my lifestyle, my choice. I could have been the poster child for healthy living over fifty.

My reward? A blood pressure that's 110 over 60.

Thanks to genetics, I never had to worry about my weight. Also, thanks to genetics, I was one in a million silent victims headed for disaster. Never saw it coming.

I had none of the classic symptoms for a stroke, except that my mom died from one. I was fifty-two years and nine months when it happened to me. It left me totally paralyzed on my right side, unable to talk, walk, or see straight.

Make no mistake about it; lifestyle does play a key role in recovery, other than that? It's a God thing.

PART ONE

THE RACE AGAINST TIME

CHAPTER ONE

THE PROMISE

I MADE A PROMISE TO MYSELF when the original narrative of *Trapped Within* was penned twenty-two years ago that I would stay true to the events and emotions of the story as they happened. But by doing so, I discovered those who read the first three chapters were literally in a state of shock by the time they finished! I've been asked on more than one occasion: *How on earth could you have done what you did?*

If this were fiction, people would have accepted what was written as part of the plot and continued reading, waiting for the next plot twist—no questions asked. But this is a true story, and that in itself commands me, as the author, to craft it in a respectful way.

As an adult who is now thinking clearly, I've asked myself the same question: *How could I have done that?* The answer is: *I don't know.* My behavior was certainly out of character for the way I normally respond. I'll be eternally grateful that no one was injured. As someone who was in the throes of a stroke (more accurately, a bleed) occurring deep within the brain, I'd say, "I tried to do my best and believed my choices were those of a reasonable person in the midst of a traumatic ordeal." I would also say, "DON'T LET ANYONE, INCLUDING YOURSELF, DO WHAT I DID!"

The story is written from the point-of-view of a person who experienced a major brain injury. It's a story few live to tell. Two out of four who have endured a bleed die immediately. One dies within a few days. One lives, but with no assurance as to the quality of their life.

Many books start with "once upon a time." One in particular began with "It was a dark and stormy night." This one begins with...

CHAPTER TWO

SUDDENLY, LIFE CHANGED

LIFE. IT FELT LIKE an extended vacation of sunny days and balmy breezes, but it was time to settle into a new routine, one that included work. The past six months had been a whirlwind with Bill's retirement, our move to Florida, and settling into a new home and community.

I was excited to return to Tropicana's executive offices. It was the second time I'd been there this month on temporary assignment. I liked everything about corporate life—the creativity and inventiveness, the brilliance of the people, the challenges, even the dress code. I wore my favorite outfit, a dark navy jumpsuit. It was dressy enough to be considered professional, yet plain enough to pass for Florida dress casual.

This time, my job was filling in for an employee in the marketing research department. I'd been a temp up north for sixteen years and worked my way up to management in a Fortune 500 company, which pretty much assured me plum assignments.

I waited as the HR coordinator finished scribbling notes in her organizer before we took the back steps to the second-floor executive suites.

"I remember you," she said with a smile. "Sonja still talks about you."

"That's nice to hear," I replied. "She made my stay here enjoyable. I learned a lot from her."

"You're going to be working with Ron this time. You remember our procedures and protocol from the last assignment, right?"

"Yes."

"Good," she said as she lightly tapped on his office door before opening it. "Look who's here!"

He grinned from ear to ear. "Now I can relax," he said.

Ron was a tall, thirty-something man with a charming smile and serious personality. He'd earned respect from his peers and colleagues by being a team player and innovative thinker.

"Ron's involved in an all-day training session with twelve execs from Chicago," Jennifer said. "So, basically, you're on your own."

I settled into the secretary's cubicle, read the neatly scrawled notes she'd written, refreshed my mind as to the computer programs she used, and braced myself for whatever challenges faced me for the day. There was one major project that needed corrections before a ten o'clock meeting. Other than that, it was quiet until lunchtime.

It was nearly noon when I decided to take a five-minute comfort break before the lunchtime rush.

When I returned to the cubicle, Ron was rustling through papers on the desk until he found a bright yellow form. He closed his eyes and shook his head.

Wouldn't you know it, I thought as I returned to the cubicle.

"What's up?" I asked.

"Did Helen leave any instructions for this?"

"For what?"

"The lunches for today's meeting."

I glanced at the note. "Not a word."

"Ah, jeez," he said with a look of despair. "We have no food and thirteen hungry people!"

He paced a few steps in front of the desk, still shaking his head, but this time mumbling.

"I tell you what—go back to the meeting," I said with confidence. "I'll get the box lunches ordered and pick them up."

He stopped. A look of questioning lingered on his face.

"It's five minutes down the road," I said with a brush of my hand. "I'll stop by HR and tell Miss Jennifer what we're doing. It'll be okay."

With a little coaxing, Ron headed down the hall.

I waited for the deli manger to answer the phone, trying to compose my thoughts. I was calling at the height of the lunch-hour crush and asking for thirteen meals to be ready in half an hour. This was asking a lot.

"I don't know if I can do it," Geo said after I explained Ron's plight.

I could hear the din of diners and clatter of plates in the background.

"I'm shorthanded."

"I know this isn't normal. Geo, I'm sure your extra effort will be well remembered. You know how much Tropicana appreciates your food and service."

He hesitated. I thought I was gaining ground until he said, "I need approval from the department head."

"He's not here at the moment," I replied.

"No approval, no sandwiches." I could hear the smile in his voice. I'm sure he could hear the surprise in mine.

I took a deep breath, thought about my options, and calmly said, "I'll have someone from HR call you. Meanwhile, we're wasting valuable time. If you start making the lunches right now, I promise I'll find the right person to approve the order. I'll see you in half an hour," I said cheerfully. "Bye." I hung up before he could find another reason to stall.

The visitor's staircase, leading from the executive suite on the second floor to the reception area on the first, curved in an arc reminiscent of an antebellum mansion. Low-backed, leather captain's chairs and glass-topped tables were clustered into conversation pits for those waiting for an appointment with staff in human resources on the first floor or executives from above.

I quickly descended the stairs and looked for the receptionist.

"Christie, have you seen Miss Jennifer?" My hand rested on the doorknob leading to her office.

"No, ma'am, they're all at lunch."

I felt a knot settle in my stomach.

"Do you know when they'll be back?"

"Not until one thirty."

"Do you mind if I leave her a note?"

She shook her head as she answered one of the three ringing phones on her desk.

The corridors to the cubicles in HR were deserted. Lights were dimmed to save energy. Except for a low-level hum from the electronic equipment, it was quiet. Spooky quiet. HAL from the movie *2001, A Space Odyssey* quiet. A radio softly played music from the forties in a far-removed cubical. No human in sight.

I raced back up the stairs, two at a time, took a deep breath, and knocked on the conference room door. I heard Ron excuse himself. The door opened and we talked in hushed tones in the hall.

"If I may use your corporate card, I'll be able to get your lunches," I said. "It will make a mess of paperwork, but we'll worry about that later. I'm going to try, one more time, to find someone in human resources who will call in the approval before I leave. I'll see you back here in about half an hour, with the food."

The deli was two miles from the office. I showed up much earlier than expected, but to tell the truth, I was too nervous to sit at the office and wait. I picked up a local beach paper and began flipping through it, not really reading anything in particular, just browsing to pass the time. The pages were filled with fishing and surfing news and bikini ads. I could hear Geo's crew frantically making lunches. I felt bad for putting so much pressure on them. Every few minutes, another white box appeared on the countertop.

"Your lunches are ready," Geo said as he pointed to the mound of white boxes. They formed a barricade between him and his customers.

With a smile of gratitude, I responded, "Phow huch mah youp flepugh?"

I could hear myself speaking. It was as though my tongue were possessed. This wasn't me!

The manager's eyes widened as the gibberish poured from my lips. I cleared my throat and tried again. Still totally unintelligible.

I handed him the credit card. He handed me the receipt and three of the boxes. As I walked to the car, my knees buckled. Before I could fall, I steadied myself on the fender. I knew at that point, without a doubt, I was having a stroke. I don't know how I knew or why I knew—I just knew. I was grateful that two of the employees brought the rest of the lunches to the car. They loaded everything into the trunk.

I blew them a kiss because I had no voice to say thank you. I got in the car and began the drive back to Tropicana. My left hand stayed on the steering wheel, but my right hand slid to my side and dropped to the seat.

There was no pain. There was no fear. All I wanted was enough time to drop off the lunches, get to the hospital, and tell my husband one last time how much I loved him. I knew I was destined to die.

CHAPTER THREE

SECONDS COUNT

I've always been one to remain calm in an emergency. When my mind goes into overdrive, I assess a situation and, within seconds, form contingency plans with safety first, then action. Driving back to Tropicana seemed like the most logical choice at the time. Thirteen blocks—turn right, four more blocks—turn right, a straight run past the wrought-iron gate, down the tree-lined driveway, and stop at the large double doors.

I took a deep, cleansing breath. *Breathe slowly,* I reminded myself, *in through the nose, out through the mouth.*

Wadda ya think, you're having a baby? I chided. My inner voice yelled, *Just breathe!*

"Huh," I snorted. *Seems like a reasonable plan.*

I wondered what I'd do if I really were in dire straits? *Lady, it doesn't get much worse than this!*

Focus, my mind repeated in a calm mantra.

I stayed in the lane closest to the curb. The iconic, twenty-acre Red Barn Flea Market was a huge tourist attraction for Bradenton, Florida, until last week when a catastrophic fire reduced the buildings to rubble. Plan B was to drive onto the open field if I lost control.

Somebody will eventually find me rising from the ruins.

The stoplight was red at Twenty-Sixth Avenue. I slowed, hoping it would turn green before I got into the mix of traffic.

It's okay, I tried to reassure myself. *It's only seconds.*

"Seconds count when having a stroke," I chanted over and over, moving my lips like a mime so I didn't have to hear the garble spilling from my mouth.

"Turn green!" I shouted at the light as though that would hasten the action. I couldn't point at it for drama like a conductor looking for a crescendo. I picked up my right arm with my left hand, turned the right hand to grip the steering wheel, and willed it into place.

"Stay!" I begged and watched in stunned silence as the paralyzed hand bounced off the console and onto the seat, settling next to my side. I could no longer feel my fingers.

People were entering and exiting Tropicana's headquarters with that corporate stride of purpose. Did you ever notice the higher the position, the longer and slower the gait? That silly thought quickly passed as I realized: *I may not be able to walk at all.*

Please, God, give me strength.

I opened the trunk, grabbed a couple of boxes, and walked towards the two-story, tinted glass doors. A young man heading for the office stopped to help and carried in the rest.

My eyes turned heavenward and I mouthed a quiet "Thank you."

Twenty-four steps on the antebellum staircase led from the atrium-styled lobby to the executive suites above. *If Ron and the rest are hungry enough, they can come get the boxed lunches themselves.*

I really don't feel well.

Seconds count when having a stroke became the din in my mind over all thoughts and conversations. I picked up the courtesy phone at the far end of the receptionist's counter and called home.

"Hello?" The sound of Bill's voice brought an immediate flush of relief. He was my rock.

"Hi, honey," I slurred. "I'm sick. Meet me at the hospital." This was the message my mind tried to convey. What Bill heard resembled words shredded like confetti.

After an eternity of silence, he responded, "I'm sorry. I think you have the wrong number."

"Nooo. No! No! No!" I shouted and began to cry.

I turned my back to avert the gaze of those in the lobby who heard the outburst.

I had to say something only he and I would know. What . . . what? What! My jaw tensed as my stomach rolled. *THINK!*

"October nineteen," I blurted out.

There was an audible gasp. "What's the matter with you?" he asked, concern edging his voice.

I took a deep breath and concentrated on forming every vowel and consonant. The words came out thick and slowly. "I'm sick. Meet me at the ER," I said and hung up. It never occurred to me that our community has two hospitals. I never told Bill which one.

There were two truths at that moment. First, time was of the essence if I hoped to survive. Second, if an ambulance came and people gathered round, it would cause a scene. I hate gawkers! What if I cursed like a sailor who'd dropped an anchor on his foot? I would be embarrassed beyond relief! It never occurred to me they'd never understand what I was saying anyway.

I considered the options:

- Call 911: I looked at the car parked in front of the building. It was steps away. The engine was still running.

- CALL 911: People now filled the lobby as lunchtime waned. I liked the employees at Tropicana. I wanted to be asked back, if I survived this crisis. The hospital was less than a mile away. There was plenty of open land.

I decided to go for it.

CHAPTER FOUR

I THINK I'M HAVING A STROKE

I PULLED INTO THE hospital's massive campus and slowly made the loop around the ER's parking lot. Not one open parking space. Not one, except in the NO PARKING zone reserved for ambulances only. My heart was beating through my chest, not because I was sick, but because I was about to break the law—me, who uses turn signals in our driveway at home. Parking in this forbidden spot was crossing the line. Driving to the hospital in the throes of a stroke seemed rational to someone with an addled brain. Charging into a reserved parking space? Not so much.

I did it, against what little good judgement I had left. I pulled in and turned the car off like I owned the place. This act of defiance made me feel like a character from the cast of *Grease*. I would have snapped my fingers if I could've still moved my hand.

It took a moment to get my balance after I slid out of the car. I leaned on the door with my right side as I locked it with my left hand. I caught sight of my face in the rearview mirror just as the security patrol cart pulled alongside me.

"Lady, you can't park here," the officer said with authority. "It's for ambulances only."

I turned and looked at him and watched his expression shift from horror to curiosity. My shoulder slumped as dramatically as a Colorado ski slope. My arm and hand swung freely with no purposeful direction, and the right side of my mouth appeared to sag and melt like a timepiece in a Salvador Dali painting.

"I think I'm having a stroke," I slurred.

He began to back his cart away, and with the professional countenance of a Deputy Barney Fife from *the Andy Griffith Show*, he said, "Don't worry about your car, sweetie. I'll keep an eye on it for you."

"Thank you" is what I'd hoped to say but remained silent.

A little help to the door would've been nice.

I watched him roll away in his specially marked golf cart. Ironically, his leaving made me think this situation may not be as bad as it seemed.

I took twenty robotic steps to the hospital's ER entry. The large double doors opened automatically with a loud whoosh of air. Apparently, the man behind the counter heard this entrance song many times before. He continued writing his notes. Eventually, he glanced at me over the stack of papers on the corner of the nurse's desk positioned between us. He blinked his eyes in disbelief.

I was beginning to feel weird. I felt as though I were standing next to myself in the middle of the foyer. I said, one last time as loudly as possible, "I THINK I'M HAVING A STROKE!"

The nurse, who was standing with her back to me, twirled around and in a hoarse whisper blurted out, "She *walked* in here?"

I stood frozen in place as faceless people came running towards me from every direction. A chatter of calls rang out over the intercom—Code Blue! Code Blue!

Someone gently rolled their arms under mine, and as my legs collapsed, this stranger lifted me onto a gurney. A sense of euphoria filled my body and blinded my senses. One tear plummeted from the corner of my eye. I sighed with relief. I made it.

The cart ride from the hospital's entrance to the exam room transported me into an unfamiliar dimension, one farther from the everyday reality we all know and live.

The aide wheeled me through dimly lit halls. Recessed lights in the ceiling blurred into a steady cadence of white flash to shadow. A bockety wheel on the gurney sent a vibration through the rubber mattress. I felt like a living rap song. Three counts of metal clatter, one beat of silence. I began to beat a four/four rhythm with my wedding band on the handrail and tried a "Pffft," but all that happened was my tongue periodically stuck out of a grotesquely shaped face.

"Are you okay, ma'am?" the aide asked.

I nodded and closed my eyes.

We passed the long waiting room. Most of the seats were filled with the sick and injured. Mothers rocked children flushed with fever in an effort to comfort them. Some patients held gauze on open wounds to slow the bleeding. Others paced, worry etched on their faces. A few gurneys lined the walls in the hall and a nurse moved from patient to patient, assessing their needs. My aide whisked me toward a private room.

A parade of professionals streamed in and out. It didn't occur to me that my vision had begun to blur. I was just curious as to how many sets of ears a doctor needed to listen to my heart with the four stethoscopes draped around his neck.

I closed my eyes and waited for Bill. It felt like it had been forever since I called him. What if he came and I wasn't in the room? Would he leave? What if I were asleep? Would he wait? What if he didn't recognize me? I'd begun to drift in and out of consciousness.

It felt like I should have been in a state of panic. Instead, I realized my whole being was in the hands of a gifted medical staff, and my spirit was with God. There were no palpable thoughts, just an aura of serenity and a longing for my husband.

"Hey there," Bill said as he pulled the curtain next to the bed back far enough to let himself in.

"Hey," I answered. "I'm sorry."

"For what?" he asked.

"I don't know." I laughed. Tears cascaded in sheets down my cheeks.

My husband's gorgeous blue eyes sparkled when he smiled. He bent over and gave me a tender kiss.

"I love you," I mumbled.

"I love you more," he whispered in my ear and hugged me tenderly.

Now I could die in peace. After all, my mother had.

CHAPTER FIVE

NO GUARANTEES

THE HOSPITAL ROOM WAS quiet, except for a monitor drumming a beat that mirrored the one in my heart. Red and blue lines on the correlating graphs jumped up and down like a bad financial day on Wall Street.

Bill's head rested on the bed, tucked in the crook of his arm. His free hand snuggled under mine.

A light tapping on the door startled him awake. The newspaper on his lap slapped to the floor and spread out like we were waiting for a new puppy to join us. I continued to sleep, unaware of my surroundings or the events that brought me to this point.

A man in a white lab coat extended his hand to Bill. Bill partially rose to greet him, but the doctor motioned for him to sit.

"How's our patient doing?" he asked in a hushed tone. "She's been sleeping since we got into the room," Bill explained.

"That's a good thing," the doctor said. He fingered the stethoscope around his neck. "I wanted to update you on our findings."

Bill buried his face in his hands for a moment before facing the doctor.

"Our test results indicate she suffered a hemorrhagic stroke, the type we more commonly refer to as a *bleed*."

Bill eyed him blankly.

"Most strokes begin when a blood clot settles in a vein somewhere in the brain and cuts off the flow of oxygen. There's a new drug that could have been administered to her if she had come to us by ambulance. It would have dissolved the clot, if it had been a blood clot. She may have had minimal, residual weakness, which could have been strengthened with physical therapy, or she may have suffered no side effects at all."

"Why are you telling me this?"

"Because this stroke is different."

"How?"

"It's a tear that was found in a weakened wall of the vein. Hers is deep within the brain in an area called the *thalamus*. Theoretically speaking, if they had administered this new miracle drug, she would have died. She's one lucky lady."

Bill sighed. "Is that why she drove herself to the hospital as sick as she was?"

"She wouldn't have been able to tell what type of stroke it was by the symptoms she was experiencing. She probably did what she did because the pressure of the stroke on that part of her brain definitely affects her ability to reason logically. Any way you look at it, her actions saved her life."

The doctor tapped his fingers on the window ledge

where he was sitting. He looked out to the Manatee River and watched a powerboat head towards the gulf.

"The bad news is, it's in an inoperable area," he said. "Unfortunately, she's going to have to fight this one on her own. I'm so sorry."

"Is she going to survive?" Bill asked.

"It's too soon to tell."

"Will she be crippled?"

"We won't know the answer to that for a while."

"What did you call it?"

"A bleed."

"No. Where it's located."

"The thalamus. It's a walnut-sized gland that controls our behavior. In fact, it's the same area of the brain that's affected by alcohol. She'll not have any inhibitions for a while."

Bill began to laugh hysterically.

Dr. Miller looked at him oddly.

"I'm sorry," Bill said. "My wife's never had a drink in her life, except for a few sips of a sloe gin fizz when she turned twenty-one."

"Cheap date, eh?" the doctor said with a sardonic smile.

"I'm a lucky man," Bill said and clasped my hand. Tears began to well. "A lucky man, indeed."

PART TWO

ADJUSTING TO LIFE

IN REHAB

CHAPTER SIX

TEFLON DAZE

I CAN'T TELL YOU when I became aware of my surroundings. Only snippets of people and incidences stuck in my mind like love bugs fused to a car's grill. The topics I clung to had no relevance to our everyday world or the way we, when healthy, perceive reality.

Time was irrelevant. Days and weeks became a mesh of rituals set by staff schedules, punctuated by doctor's appointments and family visits. It's not that I didn't look forward to any of it; it's just that I literally lived in the moment.

The past resided in a fog of shrouded memories. I could feel the emotions of an event, but visualizing the details was like trying to capture the wind between your fingers. Just like a soap bubble that floats whimsically through the air before it bursts and fades into oblivion, so did names, dates, and places that identified me as me.

The present became a never-ending cycle of Teflon moments, none sticking longer than a few hours. The good news about short-term memory loss is you can listen to the same dumb joke over and over and still laugh just as hard because everything old is new again. The bad news is, if Bill or the staff rolled me a few feet from familiar surroundings, all markers of place and space, such as doorways, hallways, signs, and décor, fused into a panorama of sameness. My mind could not grasp the subtle features that make objects unique. I had no sense of measurement. A foot, a yard, or a mile were all the same in distance.

I sensed my *self* being swallowed by this illusion and feared I'd become a reflection, a shadow of someone who once was. In the minds of others, I'd be a wisp of thought pondered for a nanosecond and dismissed. I did *not* want to morph into that reality, and without the ability to express myself and without a friendly face by my side, panic ruled my days.

Months and years or the concept of future were beyond comprehension.

When the senses are impaired and a fragile mind searches for glimpses of normalcy, repetition and ritual strengthen it. More importantly, kindness, courtesy, and respect become the building blocks towards healing.

The treatment I received at the hospital and rehab center reminded me of a morning ritual Bill has performed every day since our first day of marriage. Every morning he kisses me good-bye on the top of my head while I blissfully sleep. Sometimes I mumble "I love you." Once, while in a dream state, I gave him a bloody nose, but most often, I lay there, seemingly unaware of this sweet gift, a gift I had grown to expect. Even as I lay somewhere between sleep and awake, my senses told me whether he kissed me or not.

For example, one morning during a blizzard, when we were living north of Chicago, I heard the front door close. I sat bolt straight in bed. Unbeknownst to me, Bill had gone to warm the car before saying good-bye.

My point is, when there's deviation from ritual, it's known. I couldn't prove to you when it happened, but I knew in my gut when it didn't.

Such was the case with the beautiful, young woman standing in the doorway of my room.

"Mrs. Glim?"

"Yes," I answered with a question in my voice. I tried to focus on her face, but the light was behind her and silhouetted her body. She moved to the far, windowed wall and no closer. Something was wrong, but I couldn't rationalize what.

That little voice inside kept reminding me, *She's not your friend.*

I knew I should do something. But I didn't know what.

My mind whispered the child's slogan, *Stranger . . . Danger!*

"I have some papers for you to sign," she said softly. She didn't move.

Who is she? I wondered. I lapsed in and out of reality.

Behave, Joanie, I heard my mother say. *I raised you to be a good girl. Do the right thing.*

"I just have a few forms for you to sign," she repeated. Her voice was melodic but dishonestly off-key.

What did she want? A chorus of "stranger danger" whispered deep within my being. *Why can't I think this through?*

"I can't see to read them," I told her.

"That's okay. I'll get a nurse to help us."

I knew I had to be kind. She was a guest in my room. If I was rude, they may ask me to leave! Where would I go? Fear and confusion constricted my chest, making it hard to breath.

A dark-haired woman in a nurse's uniform joined the stranger. They stood at the end of the bed, talking in hushed tones.

I wished my husband was there. He was always by my side. *Why isn't Bill here now?* Fragments of memory shot through my mind like the flash of a strobe light, but nothing formed into a complete thought.

"It's okay," said the nurse. "Go ahead and sign it."

I took her word for it. I had to.

What if I said no? Would they punish me? Would they throw me out on the street? I pulled the blanket closer to my chest. *How would Bill find me?*

The stranger stepped forward.

"I can't write, you know," I slurred.

"Your mark will do," she replied. Her long hair covered the side of her face as she bent forward and handed me the pen. She seemed so important, dressed in a business suit and all.

"Okay," I answered reluctantly.

She never raised her eyes as she slipped the papers into her briefcase and left. Not even a thank you, a good-bye, or have a nice day.

CHAPTER SEVEN

IF TRUTH BE TOLD

I DREADED TWILIGHT SETTLING into the room. It signaled the end of another motionless day with hours spent propping my right arm up at the elbow on a cradle of pillows. No amount of concentration, therapy, or prayer lifted my hand. The fingertips pointed south like a dowser's rod looking for water. Day after day, my prayers for healing were sealed with the salt of my tears.

Except for the occasional squishing of a nurse's foam-soled shoes on the tile floor, or the occasional groan from some poor soul down the hall, everything was quiet in the evening in a rehab center. The only visitors left were the unwelcomed shadow dancers of depression and despair sliding across the floor and into the pleats of the room's partitioning curtain as the last golden rays from the sun paled and disappeared. Oh, how I hated this time of day.

"Please, God," I'd mouth into my pillow, "end this agony—if not death, then sleep."

I welcomed sleep; the cycle with no boundaries. I was whole and at home, if only in my dreams. It became my place of refuge. I could run and jump and dance. I ate without choking. I laughed and held a decent conversation. People understood what I said. I could reach and touch and grasp things in my hands. There were no limits, unless I awakened.

"Did you need something, Mrs. Glim?" the night duty nurse asked.

"I have a headache," I said through gritted teeth.

"How bad?" he asked. His arm reached above the bed and turned off the call button. "The meds cart will be around in about an hour."

"It's like a reggae band marching on Fat Tuesday!"

He brought the medicine. Within fifteen minutes, the drumming became a manageable rat-a-tat-tat and sleep transported me back to freedom.

⌒

Morning in a rehab center starts before the roosters begin to crow.

"Good morning, Mrs. Glim," the phlebotomist whispered. She snapped her finger repeatedly on the crook of my left arm's elbow to get the vein to plump. I turned my head to the right when the needle found its mark and let out a sigh when she loosened the rubber tourniquet.

"Yikes!"

"What?" the startled technician responded. Her eyes darted around the room. She held the labels for the five tubes of blood tightly in her hand. "Did I drop something?"

"Nooooo. Not that…My right arm's missing" was all the information I shared. I wanted to add, "You know the one. It's attached to a swollen and twisted hand that doesn't respond to visceral commands," but I couldn't. The look of panic in my eyes revealed a frantic search for the right word from a brain on pause. The filter allowing speech to pass from thought to formed sentence was damaged. Try as I might to access my vocabulary stockpile, the words did not materialize, so I chose silence.

"It's underneath you," said the charge nurse. She was making her final rounds before the morning shift change. "Let's get you comfortable." She rolled me on my side to face the windows. "It'll be light soon. Another beautiful sunrise is coming."

She pulled my arm away from my back and placed it on my belly.

"Do you need anything else before I go?"

"No thank you," I answered. I could hear the breakfast cart rolling down the hall. I closed my eyes and, again, surrendered to sleep.

~⌇~

It's near impossible to see God's blessings in the midst of suffering. Without recourse, my whole life had suddenly been dramatically altered. I was no longer the person I had been. The days passed into weeks and I began to realize, if truth be told, this institution may be my destiny.

CHAPTER EIGHT

TRY, TRY AGAIN

"EIGHTY-NINE POUNDS?" THE AIDE relayed to the nurse and shook her head.

"Girl, we've got to fatten you up! I weighed more than that when I was born."

Sophie, a jovial, middle-aged woman with a million braids in her graying hair, always had a smile. "Do you like it?" she asked, pointing to her hairdo. "My granddaughter wants to be a beautician. Who knows, next week she may talk me into dying it purple."

She turned slowly, and I nodded my approval.

I sat in the oversized leather chair with wooden armrests and watched her change the linens on the bed. I couldn't wait to crawl back in. All the movement from eating breakfast, washing up, and the assessment rounds left me exhausted. It made the thought of resting on clean sheets sound better than a luxury trip on a cruise ship.

"If this place fed me more than Jell-O and beef broth ..."

"Are you still choking on food?" Sophie asked.

"Yes." I nodded, thought about it, then shook my head and said, "No."

Her belly shook as she rolled her head from side to side. "Lawdy, girl!"

"I get creamy stuff now."

"It's just a precaution for a little while, honey. We don't want you to get pneumonia from inhaling a piece of food."

I shrugged my good, left shoulder. The right one slumped and twisted forward.

Sophie pointed at my right arm hanging off the side of the chair. It was her signal to me to pay attention. It's a 24-7 ordeal keeping a rogue limb and swollen-be-yond-recognition hand on my lap and out of harm's way. The whole right side of my body was paralyzed and void of feeling from my shoulder to my foot.

I had no balance front to back and limited balance to the right. I couldn't read. Print on a page was one big blur of black on white, and as long as I wore the patch on my eye, the multiple images were gone. I spoke with an eight-beer slur. It didn't matter if you understood me. I had to talk, nonstop—to anyone, anytime, any-where. Half an hour later, I'd have no recollection of the conversation.

This was my new reality. A far cry from the once dy-namic and curious person I knew me to be.

My right foot dragged behind me when Sophie as-sisted in turning me the two steps from chair to bed.

She gently lifted me onto the mattress, turned my legs, and covered me with a light blanket.

"Is Mr. Bill on his way?"

"Yes."

"Did you drop your toothbrush again?"

"Yes."

"Where did it roll this time?"

I pointed to the toilet.

"I'd ask for a new one, too!" she said with a shudder. "How many times?" She counted on her fingers. "Twelve?"

I nodded. I wished I could tell her that my time between drops was getting longer: one motion—up; one motion—down; one motion—*shit*, on the floor again.

"You've got to get those fingers moving and make a fist. I know you're praying for that. I am, too, honey," she said through the closed bathroom door. "Between us, we've got this covered, ya hear?"

"I'm working on it!" I yelled back.

I stared at my frozen fingers and sighed. It seemed futile to try again, but try I did, even though my heart wasn't in it. *Will anything make a difference?* I doubted it.

Willing it to respond didn't work. Commanding it out loud while physically changing the position of the fingers was futile. After weeks of trying, I was running out of ideas. But then I started thinking about some of the vocal techniques we used when I worked at the radio station. This brought back memories of exercises we did to make the voice more pleasing, give it more of an edge of authority. What if I changed the register of my voice, not only my speaking voice, but the voice within my head? Would that prompt a response?

I thought of my mother-in-law, who was also aphasiac. Someone suggested we encourage her to sing her words instead of saying them. It helped people who stuttered, so why not? She knew all the songs from the forties and fifties. When she heard them on the radio, she'd sing along with no problem. Bill and I began singing our conversations with her in the car. It made for some pretty funny caterwauling on the roads, but you know what? It began to work, unless we became too silly and her concentration was broken.

Maybe this idea would transfer the thought process for speech to a different part of the brain and prompt a physical reaction. Anything was worth a try. I wasn't hopeful, but I grew up in a household of inventors, so most conversations began with *what if?* I already knew the answer to *what if* if I didn't.

My gaze was riveted on the fingers. Like an athlete mentally preparing for the big moment, I calmly visualized the outcome.

"Wiggle," I said in a lower, soothing register and waited.

Nothing.

I did not avert my eyes nor raise my voice.

Please, God, help me, I pleaded.

"Wiggle," I repeated.

The middle finger quivered ever so slightly. Surprised, I blinked.

I took a deep breath, and as I slowly let it out, I repeated the command. It did it again.

"Sophie!" I screamed. "Come here, Sophie!"

The door to the bathroom flew open. Bottles of cleaning product rolled in front of Sophie as she ran to my side. "Are you hurt?"

"No," I said with a laugh. "Watch."

I looked at my hand as though in a trance.

"What am I looking at?" she asked.

"Fingers."

Just as I said that, the middle finger of my right hand raised about a quarter inch, then returned to its stagnant pose.

Sophie inhaled a gasp of air and squealed as she danced to the doorway. "Miss Jo Ann just gave me the finger!" she yelled toward the nurses' station. Her announcement was greeted by applause and running feet.

Wearing a Cheshire grin, Sophie waved her hands skyward. "Thank you, Jesus!" she shouted and danced back to my bed.

"I have to tell you, I don't usually give people who flip me the bird a hug, but in this case, I'm making an exception."

CHAPTER NINE

ON THE COUNT OF THREE

DANNY, A BIG, LUMBERING guy with a shock of red hair and the kindest, greenest eyes, spoke with an ever-so-slight brogue. Everything he said sounded either like a blessing or a curse.

"Top of the mornin'," he said with a raised brow. He tapped the glass on his watch as though the mechanism may have stopped. It was eight in the morning, and I was still in my pajamas.

"Breakfast trays were late this morning," I answered.

"Ahhh! They were still burnin' the toast when I got here," he replied with a laugh and a wink. He lifted the warming lid covering my plate, grimaced, and pointed at my silverware.

"May your tongue swallow before your taste buds realize the trick that fork played on your belly."

I rolled my eyes, dabbed the sides of my mouth, and laid the crumpled napkin on the tray.

Danny piled my hung clothing across the wheelchair's seat. With all the hangers draped to one side, the mass began to look like a technicolored centipede. "Moving day, eh?"

The nurse popped her head in the doorway. "I see you're just about ready to go. Let me get some help so we can transfer you."

"What's the matter?" Danny asked when he saw my tears.

"I wanted to tell Sophie I'd washed my face by myself this morning. It was actually more a stiff-fingered sweep up my cheeks, but . . ."

"But the point is, you did it yourself." He grinned. "It's her day off, ya know. She'll be back in the morning. She'll know where you are. Everybody knows Cody's room."

"Is she older than me?"

"Cody?"

I nodded.

"No. She just turned thirty. She's been with us for ten years."

"Oh my! She could be my daughter. What happened?"

"Car accident."

"Her body's banged up, but that doesn't keep her grounded. She goes everywhere in that electric wheelchair of hers. Watch your toes, though. She's a pretty bad driver." He shook his head and chuckled.

—⚬—

"Okay, Miss Jo Ann. I want you to lie still while we move you onto the gurney," the nurse instructed. The aides took their positions: two at my legs, two at my shoulders, and the nurse at my head.

"We're going to lift you up and slide you over. On the count of three."

"One."

I felt the aides wrap the corners of my sheet around their hands for better leverage.

"Two."

I thought of my sister-in-law and all the people she had transferred over the years as a surgical nurse. All the days of back pain she's endured from lifting more weight than the body should bear. I didn't want to be a burden on these four young aides, so on "Three!" I raised my torso as quickly as I could to make their eighty-nine-pound load lighter.

"Whoa!" shouted one young man trying to grab my knee as my leg wobbled uncontrollably. My arms and legs all shot up and out like an exploding firecracker suspended in midair. I felt like I had done a backward flip into a mosh pit on wheels. Hands grabbed for any body part closest to them, and they gently guided my runaway hulk onto the gurney.

"What just happened here?" asked the bewildered nurse.

"I tried to help," I mumbled sheepishly. "I didn't want you to hurt yourselves by lifting me."

I could hear the aides snicker.

"You weigh less than a hundred pounds, my dear," the charge nurse said gently. "There are five of us, which means we each carry about eighteen pounds of you."

Her hands cradled my face. "I appreciate you wanting to help," she said as she stifled a laugh, "but don't. Let us take care of you."

The aides piled the flowers and planters that had filled the room into every open space around my body on the gurney before they left. As Danny steered us down the hall to the elevator, he began to laugh. "You look like a Disney cartoon. All I see is a bunch of talking flowers. Where are you?"

I raised my hand in the midst of the foliage from a pot next to my hip. "Let's get this parade rolling before my petunias wilt," I commanded.

"I'm on it!" Danny said. He began whistling an Irish tune while his feet danced a jig. My hand appeared among the flowers, marking the time of the music in our one-cart procession.

CHAPTER TEN

MOVING DAY

"THEY'VE GOT YOU IN a really nice room, Miss Jo Ann," Danny said. "First floor, next to the pond, across from the nurse's station. I'd say its five-star living for rehab." Danny chose not to mention it was in the long-term care (like forever) portion of the facility.

He wheeled me closer to the window. There was a small concrete patio with a smattering of mismatched chairs and three round tables only a few feet from the room's window. The only thing between our room and this gathering space was a large privet hedge.

I watched a mama duck and her brood swim in and out of the cattails while Danny finished hanging my clothes. I liked being near the water. It was a source of comfort to me.

"Why don't they have at least one table with a full set of chairs?" I asked.

"Most of our residents are in wheelchairs. Very few people come to see them," he replied with a shrug. Their families started out with the best of intentions, but as lives get busy, it's harder to find the time to visit, or so it seems. So, there really isn't a need for more regular chairs. You'll see. Those who can usually meet their friends out here after dinner for a smoke."

—————

I could feel my body surrender to exhaustion that afternoon. My knees pulled into a fetal position. My paralyzed arm found a place of its own snuggled next to the curves of my body.

A tray with empty dishes from lunch lay on the bedside table waiting for pickup. Even simple, ordinary events like eating drained every ounce of strength I had.

Through half-closed eyes, I watched a tall, young woman with a bundle of freshly laundered clothes draped over her arm quietly enter the room. She slipped the items into the built-in dresser nearest the hallway door.

"Oh, hi," she said cheerfully. "I'm Karen, Cody's nurse-assistant. Have you met Cody yet?"

"No," I mumbled as I fought the forces of sleep.

"She'll be here in a minute," Karen said as she looked down the hall for her ward.

I could hear a low-level hum coming closer to our room.

"Cody, look out!" Karen cried out and disappeared from sight. Her warning was followed by a thud.

"Oooops" was Cody's only response. The metal from her wheelchair's leg rest scraped along the wall in the hallway with the sound of an ocean barge docking during rough seas.

"Jeez, Cody, when are you going to learn how to steer that thing?" Karen asked. She backed Cody up and centered the chair to come through our doorway. "Your new roommate's here."

Cody was a pretty young woman with thick, brown hair. She looked to be in her late twenties. Her body sat semi-prone in a massive, electric wheelchair.

"Hi," I said, my voice barely audible.

"Hi," she responded. "My name's Cody." She somberly looked at me for the longest time without saying a word.

She took a deep breath and blurted out, "My last four roommates died. Are you going to die?"

CHAPTER ELEVEN

NEW ROUTINE COME MORNING

SOMETHING CRAWLED UP MY NECK. NO—not some-*thing*, some*one*. *Someone's* fingers ... crawled up my neck. Cold, cautious fingers.

This is a heck of a way to wake up from a nap, I thought. I opened my eyes and gaped blankly at an overturned ID badge and two of the largest breasts to ever fill a nurse's uniform. I didn't know where to look! From my point of view, I now understood what a child sees while staring up at a Macy's Thanksgiving Day float, but I don't think the balloons have the same pungent aroma of five-dollar perfume and talc.

The nurse heaved a huge sigh as she grabbed my wrist and pressed her middle finger into the crease closest to my thumb. I had images of the coroner's report stating, *death by asphyxiation.*

"Do you feel anything?" Cody whispered.

"Hush."

The nurse turned and looked directly at me and realized my eyes were wide open and staring at her chest. Her scream was seismic. She stepped backward and began to laugh. "Cody thought you were dead. I was looking for a pulse."

"Please tell me you found it," I said.

"You have one, but I think mine stopped!" The nurse giggled nervously. "You scared me half to death."

"Cody, I told you, I plan on staying alive," I said.

"But dinner came and you didn't wake up."

"I'm very tired."

When the nurse opened the twill privacy curtain between our beds, I saw a very frightened young woman who had experienced way too much trauma at way too early an age.

"I'm awake now," I said. I tried to smile and reassure her. One side of my face curled upward. I quickly hid the drooping side under the blanket.

The twenty-year age gap between us didn't seem to make a difference to our relationship. We had a lot in common. We both spoke with a slur, laughed and cried at inappropriate moments, loved the outdoors, music, and parties, and had no inhibitions.

We made it a point to eat meals together in our room instead of in the dining hall. It felt more like sharing food with family. At night we'd have our ice cream before bedtime. Lights out came early. Daybreak came even earlier.

"I want to wear the red socks," Cody whined.

"Quiet, you'll wake your roommate," the aide fussed. "It's four thirty in the morning. Nobody up 'cept the birds 'n' us."

"It's okay. I'm already awake," I said. "Good morning, Cody."

"Good morning, Jo Ann," she said through the curtain. "Do you mind if I turn on the TV?"

"No. I'm going back to sleep anyway," I yawned.

I watched the bluish-gray images on the screen flash with every click of the remote, the sound vacillating between the cartoon network and VH1. This had become our morning ritual.

"Psssst. Cody! Are you awake?" I stretched my good leg and arm outward as far as they'd go. I could hear the morning breakfast cart rolling down the hall. It was now six fifteen, and the day was well under way. I waited for her to slide back the curtain that separated our beds.

"Yes," she said. Her fingers grasped the cloth and pulled. The metal clasps slid over the aluminum rod like fingernails on a chalkboard.

"It's time!" we said in unison.

Cody turned VH1 on as the commercial ended. We waited. It was hard to fathom what life would be like after Celine Deon's hit "All By Myself" slipped in the charts from number one. This had become our theme song. Cody turned up the volume on the television until it shook the vases of flowers on the cabinet below the set. I took a deep breath and together we croaked out, "ALL ... By ... MY ... self ..." It was all we knew of the lyrics and probably all the other patients and staff could tolerate.

"Good Morning, Jo Ann."

"Good Morning, Cody," I responded and waited for her high-pitched squeal. She never laughed. When she was happy, this sound began like the release of air from a stretched balloon and ended with an "Eeeeh!"

I began to laugh, but the weakened muscles in my throat produced a honking noise. The more I honked, the more Cody squealed. The more she squealed, the more I honked, a loud, uncontrollable, "HOONK...HOoNK...HoNK!" Trying to stifle it made it worse. It burst forth with the power of an air horn on an eighteen wheeler.

"Hey, I just saw Mick Jagger in the hall," the nurse announced as she entered our room. "He said he's looking for a couple of backup singers."

Cody squealed. I honked.

The nurse shook her head and grinned. "He said it definitely was NOT the two of you."

PART THREE

COMING TO TERMS

CHAPTER TWELVE

RECLAIMING ALL THAT'S SHATTERED

As physically impaired as I seemed to be, I understood and comprehended everything around me. Sounds were magnified, colors intensified, even conversations were crystal clear. Yet my responses were no broader than that of a three-year-old child. Words escaped me, and even if I captured one, most likely it had nothing to do with the topic at hand. All it did was leave the person I was talking to with a glazed look on their face and earned me a very condescending pat on the head, shoulder, or arm.

I was acutely aware of my environment, yet my physical limitations were not clear to me at all. My *self*-image was still based on the person I had been before the stroke. I knew I spoke with a slur. I knew my eyesight was compromised. I knew I couldn't hold objects in my right hand, but I never made the association between these disabilities. If I was looking at my hand, it was my hand that was impaired. If I stumbled and reeled from the wheelchair to the bed, it was my balance. Wherever I focused, therein was the malady, nowhere else.

My perception of life as I knew it was about to change today, dramatically. The early morning sunlight shone through the trees outside the window and formed a soft spotlight on the doorway leading into our room.

"Good morning, sweetheart," Bill said as he walked into the room. He held a paper bag filled with clean laundry, a bundle of unopened cards, a toothbrush, and a pair of gym shoes.

"Hey, sweetie!" I said and gave him a kiss. He surveyed my breakfast tray and gave me a thumb's up.

"What do you want to wear?" he asked.

"My baby blue sweats."

"I don't see them," he replied as he rummaged through my pajama drawer.

"Tch! They're hanging in the closet."

Since movement was beginning to return to my arm and leg, the therapist who worked with me in our room had taught me how to transfer from the bed to the wheelchair, which gave me more freedom than a fifteen year old with a driver's permit. But she didn't teach me what I was about to do next. I learned that all on my own. I rolled onto my stomach, set my feet on the floor, and pushed up with my arms. The calculated projection landed me in the wheelchair parked at the foot of the bed. The force of my weight on the unlocked chair made it roll towards Bill and stop just short of his feet.

"How often do we have to tell you to lock your wheelchair before sitting? What if you fell and broke your hip?"

"I won't," I said with a big grin and spun around to face the nightstand table.

"Do you want me to tell Dr. Caleb what you're doing?"

"No!" I knew she'd take my wheelchair privileges away. Bill knew it too.

"Then behave yourself," he said as he placed the outfit on the bed.

My feelings were hurt. I was convinced I could do that safely. After all those years of horseback riding, all those years of dance, I prided myself on some sense of rhythm and timing.

Bill lovingly washed my face and applied my makeup. He knew how important it was to me to look my best. After all, this was the first day of physical therapy in the actual gym.

"Are you excited?"

"Yes."

I had no idea what to expect. I imagined the thrill of meeting new people. I looked forward to working out on the equipment: stationary bike, weights, jumping rope ... well, maybe the latter in a week or two. I wanted to test my strength and endurance.

"Do you want me to go with you?" Bill asked.

"No."

He combed my hair and kissed me sweetly on the lips. "Okay, kiddo, I'll see you tonight after dinner."

"I love you," I slurred.

"I love you more." His words trailed out the door as he disappeared from sight.

It wasn't long before the transport aide came to get me. She centered me in the chair and rolled me down the hall at a slow but steady pace.

My functioning hand shielded my left eye from the sight of doorways whizzing past. The continual motion made me queasy. The other eye was covered with a white eyepatch to correct the double vision. I had no idea where I was or how to get back. I began to have second thoughts and wished Bill was still here.

"How far do we have to go?" I asked.

"Down this long hall and up the elevator to the second floor," she answered.

I closed my eyes and waited for the ride to end.

"Ta-dah!" The aide shouted as we rolled into the gym.

"Holy cow, this is huge!" I exclaimed. The therapy room was the size of a school gymnasium.

"Yeah, it's pretty cool," Amber said. "Let me take you on a quick tour. They've divided it into three parts." She motioned with a sweep of her hand. They just finished the fully functioning apartment to the left. It has everything you'll need to relearn how to cook and clean."

"Why would I want to do that?" I asked. "I thought not having to do housework anymore was one of the perks."

"The goal, Miss Jo Ann, is to get you strong enough

to make a smooth transition from institutional living to independent."

I sighed. "Independent living? I want to sit by the pool. Go out to dinner. Not dust."

An older woman sitting at the kitchen table smiled as she took a bath towel from the laundry basket and folded it neatly with one hand.

"Amber," I said as I motioned for her to come closer, "will they teach me how to fold fitted sheets?"

"Sure."

"I never could figure those things out."

She pointed to the far end of the room as she wheeled me into the main area. "Back there are the offices, but this middle third is where the magic happens."

The center of the room contained stationary bikes and low-level platforms for stretching. Game boards and upper-body exercise equipment were attached to wheelchair-high tables lining the outside wall under the floor-to-ceiling windows.

There was a wide span of space marked by two wide stripes painted on the floor. The oval stretched the full length of the gym and reminded me of a race track with no beginning and no end.

Amber parked my wheelchair near the entrance and behind a dark green line stenciled on the floor. The space easily held twenty or thirty chairs at one time. Space filled quickly. It reminded me of the cab line at O'Hare International Airport. As soon as an aide brought a patient in, a therapist processed the paperwork, explained the goals with the patient for that day, and off they'd go. Timers were set when a patient began a routine on the state-of-the-art equipment, and every ten to fifteen minutes, above the humming whir of exercise bikes was a chorus of timer *dings*. It sounded like a Las Vegas casino.

I had never been in a gym before. I thought of the therapist like a personal trainer and couldn't wait to get in motion. I said hello to the women sitting on both sides of me. Anna was an elderly woman with a shy smile and beautiful white hair. The woman to my right was much younger than either one of us and was going home in a day or two. Her jet black, shoulder-length hair kept cascading over her right eye, which caused her to flick the runaway strands into place whenever a particularly handsome therapist walked by.

I wondered which therapist would be assigned to me and began to look around the room. It was the first time I caught sight of the full-length mirrors on the far wall. Crouched between the white-haired woman and the lady with jet-black hair was a pathetic-looking creature slumped in a wheelchair, barely filling the seat.

"Oh, my Lord," I whispered. I looked down the wheelchair line, praying to God that someone other than me was also wearing an eye patch. Nope. I reached for my right arm, which was hanging limply over the side of the chair, and watched as the reflection in the mirror mimicked my every move. I couldn't catch my breath.

This was the first time I had seen my*self*, my whole self, since the stroke—except for a glimpse in a very small, blurred mirror in a dimly lit bathroom. I had no idea so much had been stripped away.

"What happened to me?" I yelled out loud and began to sob uncontrollably. "What have you done to me?"

"What's wrong?" Jim asked as he bent next to me.

I buried my head in his chest. "Please take me out of here. I can't look in the mirror."

"It's okay," he said quietly. "We'll work in the hall-way today."

CHAPTER THIRTEEN

RECALIBRATING THE BIG SIX

I SAT QUIETLY IN front of Linda's desk staring at the barren wall behind her. Boxes filled to capacity with books and mementos were neatly piled against the back wall of her new office. The petite woman thumbed through a bulging briefcase tucked between her legs.

"When the brain's been injured," the speech therapist explained, "we use everything in our arsenal to help restore it. There are many ways in which we can stimulate the senses to prompt the brain and help it heal. Identifying the objects on this stack of children's flashcards is one way," she said and deftly laced a card through her fingers with the hand of a professional dealer before shuffling the deck.

She palmed six cards to the table and neatly lined them up in front of me.

"Today, we're going to figure out how much information you've retained since the stroke."

Linda's eyes were piercing blue. She looked at me with laser-beam focus, studying every nuance of speech I may utter before I even formed a word.

"People take the big six for granted," she said. "We rely on our strongest senses, like vision or hearing, and treat the others like backup singers." She chuckled at her own joke.

"But when you've had a brain injury, sweetie," she added as she adjusted the glasses slipping to the end of her nose, "it's important to go back to basics and learn how to form speech by using all your senses."

Her hand pointed at the cards in front of me. She tapped on one in particular.

"Look at the object and tell me what you see."

My lips moved, but no words evolved. I looked at Linda through pleading eyes and blinked a thousand times as though that would find the frayed wires in my head so we could splice a new connection. Aphasia be damned!

How could life have come to this? There was a time, not that long ago, when my paycheck was directly linked to my voice. You don't get paid to pantomime on the radio.

I knew the picture was a pencil. I knew how to use it, but to name it? Hah! The words formed easily in my mind and swirled toward my mouth, but it seemed the stroke jammed a pause button somewhere between my eyes and my tongue and I was mute.

Calmly, she prompted, "Close your eyes and see yourself touching it."

I sat in silence for a moment, my hand outstretched.

"Pick it up and hold it. What's it feel like?"

My hand rolled palm up as I lifted the imaginary object.

"Did you ever put it in your mouth?"

She paused to give me time to think about it. "What did it taste like? Did it have a smell?"

I could smell the freshly sharpened wood and lead tip. My head slowly nodded.

"Think it. Say it."

"It's a p-p-p," I stammered and snorted in defeat.

"Take your time."

I cleared my throat. "It's a pen. A pen. . ." I knew that wasn't right and slapped my knee in frustration. "It's a pencil!"

Linda clapped for the pure joy of witnessing my success.

I grinned as best I could with one side of my mouth still pointing south. "More!" I shouted.

"Okay, what's this?" she asked as she pointed to the next card, and the next, and the next. Some I got immediately. Some I struggled with, and even though I was mentally exhausted by the end of the session, the response to victory was always "more."

"Do you want to take some of these back to your room and practice tonight after dinner?"

I enthusiastically nodded yes.

Linda followed my gaze to the top of her desk as we waited for the aide to return me to my room.

"Are you curious about this?" she asked.

I nodded.

"It's a book I'm reading, *Quiet Days in Clichy* by Henry Miller. He's very quotable. So far, my favorite is . . ." she paused to find the page. "Ah! Here it is."

In life's ledger, there is no such thing as frozen assets.

"That reminds me of my aphasiac patients and to me offers them a message of abundant hope. And that means you." She rested her hand on my shoulder. "Regaining speech is difficult, and for some it may never return, but as Henry Miller said, 'there are no frozen assets.' So, I want you to keep trying."

CHAPTER FOURTEEN

WHAT A MESS I'M IN

Having the stroke was easy.

I had received my once-in-a-lifetime call. It was the hour of reckoning, the conclusion of my life's journey. There was no fanfare. No bedside vigil. No time to plan or say good-bye, make amends or atone with God. This was it. My life as I had known it was over. My spirit was to be catapulted from this reality to a transcending universe known as *eternity*. It was time to return to the presence of God. There was no fear, only a sense of destiny, and at that moment, I realized I truly believed what I had always embraced, my Christian faith.

Surviving a stroke? Therein lays the struggle.

"Where's God when I need Him?" I whispered to Margi as she took my vital signs. It was midnight, one of the few hours of quiet in a rehab facility where reality and doubt collide.

"What a mess I'm in. . . What a mess I am, I am!"

She pulled a chair next to the bed and rested her arms on the mattress next to my head. "What's going on, lovey?"

"I don't understand. Why didn't God take me? You have a stroke. You die."

"Do you think he's punishing you?"

"No. I just think, for some reason, He doesn't want me." A lump formed in my throat as tears filled my eyes. I felt abandoned and alone.

"I love God more than life itself. I've lived my beliefs to the best of my abilities, but I guess it wasn't good enough."

"God didn't do this to you," Margi said. "If anything, He's helping you to heal. He's got plans for you."

My pressed lips and bowed head telegraphed my thoughts, and they certainly did not agree with Margi.

"Do you know the statistics for a bleed?" she asked. "That's the type of stroke you had."

I shook my head no. Even if someone had told me, memories do not stick to a Teflon brain.

"What happened to you was not caused by a blood clot. It was a tiny tear in a vein or an artery deep within the brain. Two out of every four patients who endure this type of stroke die immediately; one dies a few days later; and one will survive, but there are no assurances as to how able-bodied they'll be. Usually, there are very serious physical limitations. You, my dear, are slowly regaining what you have lost. It's too soon to tell how far you'll come, but you are truly a walking miracle."

I looked at my right hand, still swollen beyond recognition, the fingers now curling into my palm.

Margi cradled my injured hand in hers and began to

massage the palm and fingers with the pad of her thumb. "Do this every day," she said. "Ask Paula the occupational therapist. She'll tell you. It improves circulation."

I watched as she gently pressed into the hollow of my hand with a circular motion, then across each knuckle, and up each finger.

"I understand what you're struggling with, lovey," Margi said. "I was in a horrible car accident about four years ago. They didn't think I'd survive." Her mood turned somber. "Before I was catapulted through the windshield, my head clipped the rear view mirror. It sliced a piece of my skull clean off, right here."

She pointed to her hairline.

"At first, that gaping wound reminded me of everything I'd lost, and I was angry at God. Now, the indentation in the front of my head reminds me how lucky I am to be here."

"Can I see it?"

Margi took my fingers and pressed them over her scalp until they slipped into a triangular indentation. I could feel her heartbeat press back.

"Sometimes, it's the trauma, not the drama, in our lives that makes us stronger, but we have to be willing to strip ourselves naked to find it. No more ego, or vibrato, or attitude. It's a solitary journey to find your soul. I had no idea before the accident that I was about to embark on a physical and spiritual journey of healing. You're at the beginning of it, should you choose."

Sadness engulfed me. "I believe everything you're

saying. So, why am I having such a difficult time embracing those words for myself?"

"I have a feeling you'll find your answer to that."

"You're lucky you survived," I said as I stroked her hand. "Did being a nurse help?"

Margi turned her head toward me, her gaze met mine. "I didn't go to nursing school until *after* my recovery."

A-F-T-E-R. The word echoed through my mind. *There is life after. Not just an existence, but a life. A life altered, maybe, but still a life worth living.*

Later, as sleep pulled me closer to her darkened sanctum, I prayed:

Dear God, I don't know what you want from me. I don't know what's ahead, but I promise you this: I'll work like an Olympian to get better. If I don't, I know where I am now is where I will continue to be. If I do and I don't improve, then I'll know it's my destiny. If I improve, I know it will be through your grace. Please guide me. I need you. Thank you for all my blessings, especially my sweet hubby, Bill. Amen.

CHAPTER FIFTEEN

DON'T TELL ME
I'M STILL ME

"I'VE MADE AN APPOINTMENT for you to meet Dr. Finkle," Dr. Caleb informed me during her weekly visit. She scanned the order for the time and date. With a frustrated sigh, she snapped the chart shut. "Someone will let you know the details."

Dr. Who? Why? I wondered. It never occurred to me to ask because by the time I did, I'd have forgotten what I wanted to know. Instead I just replied, "Okay."

Dr. Caleb took my hand in hers. "I think you're having a hard time adjusting to your condition. Dr. Finkle may be able to help."

"Okay," I answered. My ever-present tears left a glistening trail on my cheeks.

How does anybody come to terms with a body you don't recognize as your own? When I drove myself to the hospital, I was whole. Now, a few short weeks later, I couldn't walk, could barely talk, and struggled to see.

The right side paralysis made it impossible to do even menial, daily tasks. Eating without someone cutting my food was impossible. Dressing was an aerobic workout that left me breathless. I had to accept assistance for everything. I grieved my loss of freedom because I was trapped within this imperfect body.

~⌒~

Cody and I had been sitting on the patio next to the water, watching a handful of exotic birds fishing near the cattails. It was a beautiful Florida night, gentle breeze, and low seventies. Cumulus clouds were saturated with amber hues from the setting sun, and a sky streaked in red and purple mirrored the heavenly scene on the surface of the pond.

"We better head in, Cody. I don't want to get locked out again. Last time, you and your chair almost ended up swimming with the fish." I reached for the button on the wall that opened the large double doors leading into the patient's recreation hall.

It was refreshing to feel the air-conditioned air on our bodies as we headed towards our room. Cody maneuvered her state-of-the-art electric wheelchair in front of me until we reached the main hallway next to the dining room.

My chair, a hospital issue, *roll-the-wheels-yourself-if-you-want-to-move* model fit perfectly behind hers. It was not unusual to see the two of us in tandem, rolling down the halls, Cody in front and me hanging on for the ride.

"Okay, I'm backing up," Cody announced over the shrill, pulsing beeps that signaled reverse. However well-intentioned, Cody's driving was atrocious!

"Cody, you're too close to me. Don't back up," I warned her, but the chair continued to move.

"Cody, wait!" Panic shouted through my voice. To see that massive battery pack and wheelchair coming at me was like watching a semi chase a tricycle. My feet pushed and slipped on the polished tile as I tried to pick up traction.

"Cody, stop!" the activities director commanded. She lifted Cody's fingers from the controls. "How's about I walk you two back to your room?"

I nodded like an over-enthusiastic bobblehead.

"Are you coming to the St. Paddy's Day party on Friday?" Carla asked.

My head continued to wobble. Cody squealed. I honked. Carla laughed.

"I'll take that as a yes." She checked our names under "attending" on her invitation sheet.

"Dr. Finkle's waiting for you in the lounge, Miss Jo Ann," said the CNA as she unlocked the laundry room door behind Cody and grabbed an armful of clean towels.

"Tomorrow's bath day, ladies!"

"Yay!" Cody and I shouted in unison.

We all said our good-byes and I rolled on down the hall.

In the past few days, I had gained enough strength and flexibility to push myself through the halls. I could now swing my right arm forward and back, a *huge* improvement. Each spin of the wheels was laborious. A shuffle of feet on the floor, a deliberate push with my left hand on the left wheel and a roll of my right arm over the other propelled me in a straight line, even if the measured distance per rotation was in inches. The lounge, five doors from my room, seemed like a mile, but I was determined to get there under my own power.

I felt a pang of apprehension as I opened the library door. I wanted this man to see me as I really was, the energetic, inquisitive, on-the-go me from before the stroke. Not this skinny shell with an ugly arm. I wanted him to see that my mind and spirit were still intact, in spite of my flickering memories. I still had all my faculties. I didn't want him to concentrate on my slurred speech or raw emotions. Positive changes were happening, slowly, very slowly.

This was a large, quiet room except for an air-conditioning unit that heaved and quaked at the oddest moments. Books, fragile from age, lined the makeshift shelves. An old piano dominated the corner of the room. A handwritten sign announced a Sunday sing-along, at ten a.m. *All are Welcome*, the sign said in embellished, handwritten script. From the looks of the hymnals, many a tune had been sung as someone plunked on those vintage keys.

Dr. Finkle sat on an oversized leather chair next to the coffee table. A floor lamp cast a dim light on the papers scattered before him. His brindled beard reminded me of my sixth-grade teacher, which is probably why I liked him as soon as we met. Mr. Vonnegut had been my first, real crush.

Dr. Finkle stayed on point. He was honest without being hurtful and funny without making light of the situation. No matter what we talked about, he kept coming back to the same scenario. One I could not grasp nor accept. Over and over again he told me, "You are still you."

"The *me* you refer to could not be further from the *me* I know," I said emphatically.

He leaned back in his chair and studied the scowl on my face.

Four weeks earlier, I was healthy—a viable commodity on the job market. I was able to ride a bike or a horse, go for a swim or out on our boat, make love to my husband, work in the garden, or drive to the store. I could do intricate needlework, paint, play handbells, and read. So, DON'T TELL ME I AM STILL ME.

Here, I sit before you, slumped in a wheelchair with a patch on my eye. My arm dangles limply at my side, an arm swollen and deformed beyond recognition. During the day it hangs off the side of my wheelchair. At night while I sleep it flops behind me and snuggles up against my back. It's never where a normal arm would be. I constantly tug at my elbow to swing my arm onto my lap. I know it's mine, but it's so grotesquely deformed from the stroke that I can't identify it as my own. So, DON'T TELL ME I AM STILL ME. This . . . is *not* me.

All it took was one catastrophic event, and I could take my resume, with all its accolades and awards and achievements and schooling, and throw it to the wind. It isn't worth the expensive paper on which it's written. So, DON'T TELL ME I AM STILL ME.

I could see the compassion in his eyes, but it did not ease the blow of his words. "You need to get used to the idea that you may not progress much further than you are right now," he said quietly. "There are no guarantees that it will get much better."

As he wheeled me back to my room, thoughts about our conversation tormented my brain like burrs under a saddle. I had expected a more positive message. "You're doing great, kid" would have been nice. "You're remarkable" would have been better. But to tell me, after all the hours of physical and speech therapy, that I was on the par of normal, and then to announce that I probably would not advance any further than I already had made me furious!

No one wants to live with false hope, but don't the answers to recovery lie somewhere within the individual? It had only been a month since the stroke. The neurosurgeon told me my window of opportunity for healing was two years, the extent of recovery unknown. Had that changed? Would I have to live with my ugly arm? Would I be wheelchair-bound for life? Would my words slur and tears flow during every conversation? Forever?

"Eventually, you're going to have to redefine who you are," he said, and as he left, he added, "You have my number."

I could feel my jaw tense. What was I willing to settle for? Would I be content to be confined? Even after all the hard work, would I have a choice in the outcome? If I chose not to work toward healing, the outcome was clear. I'd spend the rest of my life as an invalid. If I set my goals with no restrictions, then when all was said and done, I'd have to make peace with it and live with the consequences. Either way, the outcome was in God's hands. Not Dr. Finkle's. Not mine.

"I believe in miracles!" I shouted after him.

"I do believe . . ." I whispered.

"I do," I mouthed. The tears fell freely.

CHAPTER SIXTEEN

THE FACE-OFF

NANCY HANDED ME A TOWEL to wipe the sweat from my face. "You gave me fifteen minutes this morning, Miss Jo Ann. Good job!"

"I'll give you fifteen more," I said with a smile and leaned back in the seat of the stationary bike, feet slowly pedaling.

"Are you sure?" She checked my heart rate.

"I won't make it to Denver by sitting still, now will I?

"I forgot." She chuckled. "You're riding cross-country. How far are you now?"

"I can see Louisiana on the horizon," I answered. "I want to get to the state line before sunset. There's a great steak place at the far end under the bridge."

"You got it," she said and set the timer for another fifteen.

I liked to play this charade while I rode the bike-to-nowhere. I'd close my eyes and visualize the places Bill and I have seen on our cross-country travels. I out-pedaled my rehab reality in fifteen-minute increments every day. Planning my destination kept the anger and depression at bay, most of the time. At least until Nancy helped me off the bike and onto the wheelchair. I hated that chair. Even though it allowed me mobility, it was a continual reminder of what I could not do.

"Are you going to spin those wheels like you're driving a race car again?" Nancy asked.

"Maybe," I said with a shrug.

"I'm supposed to tell you not to do that," she warned with her hands on her hips.

"Maybe not." A sideways, impish grin crossed my face.

She shook her head and stifled a grin as I left the therapy room.

"See you tomorrow," I called to her over my shoulder.

"Keep it slow!" shouted the charge nurse. She pulled the med cart closer to the wall.

"I'm looking for my real arm. It's around here somewhere. Have you seen it?"

She rolled her eyes and pointed to the main corridor.

I'd formed a particular fondness for the shortest hallway nearest the facility's front entrance. It sloped from the elevator to the north/south wings about sixty feet away. An opened fire door tethered to the wall at the mouth of the southern corridor stood sentinel against all who passed by this three-way intersection. That door, in its imposing stance, became my nemesis.

One evening after dinner and before visitors arrived, I waited on the thin, black line of marble that separated the halls to the residents' rooms from the lobby. It was next to the elevator we all used to access the gym and the second-floor patients' rooms. This black line was the finishing piece for the opulent, art-deco marble floor in the reception area.

Like a downhill skier waiting for the starting pistol at the beginning of a race, I waited until all was quiet. I placed my feet firmly on the footrests of the wheelchair, set the palms of my hands on the metal rim on the wheels, and pushed. The goal? Close the fire door with the force of my body slamming into it, thereby uncoupling the manual "open" position that held the door in place.

From the starting point, the fire door didn't look that large. Gravity and momentum propelled me forward. As I got closer, the door loomed like a linebacker on the opposing team poised on the scrimmage line during the Super Bowl—unwilling to yield to any attack. I stuck my legs straight out and waited for the impact. My feet hit the door, and my body folded like a Japanese fan. The wheelchair smashed into the door with a terrible sound of steel colliding with steel. The door stood firm, but the noise from the crash reverberated down the halls. Alarmed aides and nurses came running from everywhere.

"Are you all right?"

"What happened?"

"I guess I need more practice cornering," I answered timidly and rolled towards my room.

Every few nights after dinner and before Bill came to visit, I'd repeat this ritual. This had become a Trojan door harboring all my demons and grief. It had to be defeated. I'd plan the hit, think about the results, and plot for the next battle. Because of short-term memory loss, I can't tell you how long this continued, but I do remember the last time.

I waited for the halls to clear. My hands gripped the wheels of the chair. I was ready to roll. My teeth were clenched, body rigid, eyes narrowed. I began the slow, me-thodical rhythm of grabbing the wheels from behind my back, pushing upward with the palm of my hands, and as they reached the highest point next to my body, sliding them away to let gravity increase the maximum speed.

Wisps of hair blew across my face.

The door stood tall in the shadows of evening light. The institutional beige, square tiles of flooring blurred as I picked up speed—past the elevator, down the in-cline, over the leveled area next to the bathroom entry-way. My body lurched forward. I set my heels against the impending force and prepared for the approaching launch after the second incline.

Focusing on the door, I saw my reflection in the tiny slit of window near the door's massive handle. As I drew closer, I threw my feet forward and waited. Those spin-dly legs hit the door solid. My knees did not buckle.

The massive door shuttered and groaned as the wheelchair pushed into it. The force spun me sideways in the chair and sent me and the chair careening backwards into the hallway. The fire door, ever so slowly, began to move toward me, and as I watched, it slammed shut with the kur-chunk of a jailhouse gate.

My first win. I had begun to conquer my demons.

PART FOUR

BREAKING FREE

CHAPTER SEVENTEEN

HAD ENOUGH

I PICKED AT THE frozen peas on my plate. The ones boiled to perfection, then warmed to mush. They had cooled to room temperature, not as a cuisine delicacy, but because they were the last thing I wanted to put in my mouth. The outside tine on my fork squished each orb into a mash of green paste. It didn't improve the veggie's taste or my foul mood.

"I've had enough, Cody," I said and dropped the fork onto the tray with a clatter.

"Well, at least you finished the fries."

"I'm not talking about the food," I said with a sigh. "It's hard to believe it, but it's been five weeks since I entered rehab, six since the stroke."

"What are you talking about?" she asked.

"I need something that feels normal. Like a shopping mall. I want to go shopping. See people. Feel the cloth between my fingers. Hold a charge card in my hand, for crying out loud!"

Cody stared at me with a vacant, "something's-wrong-with-what-you're-saying" kind of a look penciled on her face.

"Oh, I don't like the sound of this," she said.

"Look. I'm learning how to dress myself. Why can't we practice in the dressing room of a department store? Why do I have to continually pull on and off the same old, stretched-out sweatshirt I wore yesterday and will probably wear again tomorrow?"

"Did you tell the therapist that?"

"Yes, I did." My foot kicked at the air like a petulant child as another deep sigh rolled off my lips. "I told her it would lift my spirits and accomplish her goals, but nooooo. She's totally unmoved by what I had to say."

"What are you going to do?"

"I don't know."

The room filled with an uncomfortable silence. The only sound was Cody sipping the last few drops from her super-sized soda.

I rocked back and forth on the edge of the bed, my arms folded across my chest. "Therapy sessions are over for the day," I mumbled. "I've finished dinner. And Bill's not coming tonight."

"Where's Bill?" Cody asked.

"Choir practice." I looked at Cody with glee. "I'm going to do it!"

"Do what?"

"I'm taking myself to the mall."

"Oh, this is a bad idea. Bad, bad idea."

"Cody, it's going to be fine. It's not that far."

The light to the nurse's station began flashing outside our hallway door. I could see a hint of red shadow on the opposite wall.

"Did you just push your call button?"

No response.

"Cody, you better come up with something when they get in here." I began to panic. I knew they'd stop me if they knew. "I'll ask the nurses what they think before I leave, okay?"

"You ask. Don't just go."

I wheeled myself down the hall and slowed at the nurse's station. Margi was on shift tonight. "Cody's call is a false alarm," I said and headed towards the front of the building.

"Oh, okay," she said, never looking up from the mound of pills she was counting.

It was busy tonight. Mrs. Flanagan's family gathered in the reception area to celebrate Nana's eighty-eighth birthday. People of all ages clustered in pockets around the presents, the cake, and the old woman, but the doorway path was clear.

There were as many lights lit on the switchboard, next to the front door, as there were on the cake. The receptionist never lost her composure. The courteous tone in her voice and calm demeanor never gave any indication as to the number of demands on her attention.

I slowly rolled towards the full-glass double doors leading to the outside world. The sun was low in the sky, casting warm shades of gold around the waiting room.

An ambulance, with lights still pulsing, pulled up and parked under the roof overhanging the main entrance.

Betty was talking in hushed tones as I neared her desk. She held a cluster of wires from the switchboard in her left hand, pulling one at a time and connecting them to the appropriate room numbers on the console. The cord from the headset dangled under her chin and swayed with her body as her chair rolled from one side of the station to the other.

I nodded a hello to the receptionist as I continued toward the door. Her eyes riveted on me. Her answers to the anonymous caller (wrapped in the wire around her head) were short, one-word responses: "Okay…uh-huh…yep."

The double doors slid open, and a warm sweep of jasmine-scented air rushed in. I closed my eyes and enjoyed the fleeting moment of life beyond.

I turned my head when I heard the click of heels on the marble floor. "You're Cody's roommate, right?" Betty asked as she placed her hand on the back of the wheelchair.

"Yes," I answered. I glanced at the doors and turned back to meet her gaze.

"I thought so," she said. "We met the first day you came here."

"I'm sorry," I said and shook my head. "There's a lot I don't remember."

"I brought you that beautiful bouquet of flowers."

"Thank you," I replied, hoping for a flash of the

event, but it never happened. "That was very nice of you."

The sky was turning darker. Soon, dusk would cover us with the quilt of night shaded in purples and deep blue. Street lights began to flicker. Car lights illuminated the road, passed, and left the world once again in darkness.

I was beginning to have second thoughts about going to the mall. I didn't think to bring a flashlight. I didn't have one anyway. I really didn't know how far it was to the mall or which direction to take when I got to the road.

"I don't think you want to go out there," Betty said as she patted my hand. "The ground is very bumpy and not safe for wheelchairs."

I was mesmerized by the cord from the headset shimmying like a belly dancer. The rhythm from her double chin and the bouncing tube were quite hypnotic. The charm of her words, the movement of the tube, and the fact that people don't lie made me agreeable to stay. Besides, Mrs. Flanagan's granddaughter brought me a piece of red velvet cake. How could anyone say no to that?

Betty opened the curtains near her desk so I could enjoy the dusk settling over the entryway gardens. Twilight was spectacular as day gave way. It wasn't long before Margi came to get me.

"Okay, Bambi, let's go home," the nurse said as she wheeled me towards One South.

Bambi was a nickname I'd acquired a month before my stroke. It happened quite by accident. Being new to Bradenton, I had a first-time office visit with our insurance-appointed primary care physician. The building was in an older part of town—a rapidly changing neighborhood with residents whose names were as colorful as they were: Boom-Boom McKenzie, Caress Williams, and Squatty Sanders were the latest to make the front page of the paper (not the society section). The receptionist was going through the usual mountain of paperwork to set up the new account. She began adding our home information to her records.

"What's your name?" she asked matter-of-factly.

"Jo Ann," I answered in the same robotic cadence.

It was difficult to hear. Phones were ringing; people were talking. Someone called to her from down the hall. You could tell she was flustered and couldn't think of the word address when she blurted out, "What's your street name?"

A perplexed look and brief smirk crossed her face. She blushed and giggled as she said, "That wasn't quite what I meant to say."

"That's okay," I said with a straight face. I winked as I blurted out, "Just call me Bambi."

Tonight, after the visitors were gone and I was tucked in bed waiting for the daily, anticipated ice cream, Margi came into the room, her hands tucked behind her back.

"Here you go, Bambi," she said with a giggle and presented me with a cherry tart.

CHAPTER EIGHTEEN

THEM

WHAT FORTIFIES THOUGHTS OF worthlessness in the mind of someone recovering from a catastrophic illness? For me, it was THEM.

The THEM who could deem me miraculously cured when my ninety days of insurance coverage reached the eighty-five-day mark. Never mind I couldn't pee without someone balancing me while I was on the pot.

It's the THEM who could surmise I was no longer contributing to society, and therefore nothing more could be done to improve my condition. THEY could ship me home with little or no homecare assistance. THEIR decision could leave my family no choice but to pay for additional care beyond our savings.

This is the THEM who warehouses the feeble and ailing for the duration of their natural lives and coddles (or worse, ignores) these dear souls until they die. Sometimes a well-intentioned loved one faces serious decisions with a very heavy heart, based on the reams of records from THEM.

They are the THEM who sit in offices miles from the front lines of healthcare. THEY strap the hands of medical personnel and muffle or ignore the pleas of the patient. These are the THEM with no identity, no empathy, no association with humanity, only a passion for numbers. THEY live to count numbers, to tally statistics, to balance life in black and red ink. THEY show no mercy, or compassion, or heart. Our progress and treatment, or lack thereof, is determined by these creatures, their manipulation of actuarial tables, knee-jerk federal laws, and the person's ability to pay. And pay, we do. THEIR decisions do more to devastate self-esteem and the will to survive than could ever be imagined or measured.

THEY are the THEM with the authority to yea or nay our healthcare needs.

<hr />

"Where are we going?" I asked Bill. He pushed the elevator button for the second floor. His mood was somber and preoccupied.

"We're going to Carol's office. We have a meeting with the claims assistant at the insurance company to evaluate your condition and treatment plan."

Carol was the caseworker assigned when I arrived at the rehab center. She is a truly kind and patient person. She, along with the doctors, staff, and therapists, evaluates my charted progress and plans for future therapies depending on the chart's results. It's a team approach, and it works. Periodically, Carol has to justify my care to THEM.

I met THEM in Carol's office that morning.

"Good morning," I mouthed to Carol as Bill wheeled me next to her desk. She was already on the phone with THEM.

She looked weary as she listened to the voice.

"I see," she interjected at acceptable pauses.

She scribbled notes on an in-house pad of paper and doodled in the margin when she was placed on hold. The margin was filled with stick figures, hearts, and geometric designs indicating she'd been on hold a lot!

"The treatment's progressing nicely, but—" Her head slowly nodded. She covered the mouthpiece of the phone with the palm of her hand. "He cut me off again," she whispered and crossed her eyes.

"Yes. That's correct." She nodded. "In Dr. Caleb's estimation, it would be premature to end speech therapy."

I looked at Bill in disbelief. "They're stopping speech therapy?"

He raised his finger to his lips and leaned closer to hear Carol's one-sided conversation.

She closed her eyes and slowly shook her head. "I see." She sighed. "Well, we'll make an effort to accomplish what we can in the next few sessions this week."

She hung up the receiver and shrugged her shoulders. "I'm sorry."

"You did your best," Bill responded.

"What the heck just happened here?" I asked.

"The good news is they think you're progressing nicely," Carol said as she half-heartedly smiled at me. "The bad news is your speech therapy will be terminated the end of this week." She handed Bill the notification from the insurance company.

"My speech therapy stops because I'm recovering? Do you mean to tell me they think I'm healed?"

Bill and Carol ignored me and continued talking in muffled tones.

"Excuse me. I'm still here," I said and tapped my fingers on the end of the desk. Both heads turned and looked directly at me.

"Who the hell are THEY?" I asked. I could feel a flush of anger pulse from my neck to my face.

With no response to my question, Carol and Bill continued shuffling papers and talking between themselves.

I crossed my arms and glared out the window. My left foot kicked the leg guard on the wheelchair as though I were responding to a sibling who'd said, "Ha-ha, I told you so."

There was a time when my voice was my paycheck. My ability to communicate entertained the ears of thousands. Not anymore. The stroke robbed me of any thoughts of conversing in a professional way.

Do THEY think as long as I can grunt for food when I'm hungry and squeal when I feel the urge to pee that that's all I need to survive?

Rage turned to tears that cascaded down my face.

"Why am I being punished for doing so well?" I asked.

This was a fight for my very existence. The staff could share their professional knowledge, but if I did not commit myself like an athlete in training, I would be disabled forever. Even if I did do everything asked of me, I could still be disabled for the rest of my life. The only guarantee I had was, if I didn't try, the outcome would already be clear. I wasn't willing to accept that as the final outcome.

Every step forward elevated me to another level of competence and strength. I didn't place expectations or limits on my abilities. I'd imagine the possibilities and work diligently to achieve my own personal best. If I didn't try, I knew what the outcome would be. If I tried, I may be pleasantly surprised, or I may have to accept the fate dealt to me. It was too soon to tell which direction my life would take.

Carol pulled a tissue from the box on her desk. She handed it to Bill, who in turn handed it to me. "If THEY knew I can comprehend what I read, would my therapy have ended sooner?"

Carol shook her head and gave me an I-don't-know look.

"I know I have the potential to do everything again. I just need a little more time and guidance to make it a reality."

The social worker scribbled a note.

It's easy to become discouraged, to want to give up. Every waking hour, there's something to fight against: a body that won't cooperate; an impersonal health system trying to save money; personal demons of grief and doubt. Even on a *best* day, I was still held captive.

Sleep. Only sleep offered sanctuary.

CHAPTER NINETEEN

WHEEL INVISIBLE

I HAD COUNTED EVERY hour last night in fifteen-minute increments from lights out to dawn. You'd think I would have been exhausted, but I couldn't wait to start this day. It'd been a week of firsts, beginning with my first, hesitant steps. No assistance. No railings. No hand holding mine. Only a wheelchair trailing my backside for that planned sit when my legs gave out from exhaustion. For those efforts, I'd been awarded an institutionally issued, bright silver cane with a large, puke-colored rubber tip glued to the ground end.

Tah-dah!

Oh, how I wished for a gnarly tree-branch staff, a rod whittled with pine trees and the wildlife of a Pacific Northwest forest. The top purposely carved into a stylized star with rounded spires to offer stability for my good hand. I envisioned semiprecious gems set as the peering eyes of animals within the carved forest on this work of art. To add to the ambiance, seeds would nestle freely in the shaft, and every time the cane was raised or shaken or turned upside down, the sound would mimic gently falling rain.

That's what I wanted.

What did I get? An ugly stick! I was not complaining, only wishing. That drab metal monster pushed me closer to life as I once knew it, one shaky step at a time. For that I was grateful. I was ever nearer to the day when I could rely on nothing but my own strength to propel myself forward and expect to be in an upright position when I reached my destination.

My biggest *first* that week was yet to come. Today I'd been granted a pass into the outside world, the first since the stroke. It was a day for rejoicing, not only for me but for everyone. Today was Easter! The anticipation of this celebration filled my heart with joy and gratitude. I had survived a life-and-death struggle. The road to recovery still lay ahead, but with every small victory towards normalcy, a sense of hope filtered through like the bright rays of sun through a storm cloud.

The CNA helped me wash up and applied my makeup. Bill would be here soon, and it'd be a race to church before the crowds arrived.

"Good morning, sweetheart," Bill said as he kissed the nape of my neck. His hands were filled with cards and clothes. Twenty-four years after our wedding, and he still sent chills through me with his touch.

"Good morning," I answered, kissing him tenderly

on the lips. "Wait till you see what I can do now."

He flashed a look of hesitancy and laid my outfit on the end of the bed. "Am I going to like this?"

"Watch!"

I took the cane in my hand and stood up, humming a made-up tune. My body swayed to the impromptu melody. I tossed the cane toward my affected arm. It made a gentle arc in the air and immediately fell to the floor.

I grinned. "I don't have that part of the routine down yet."

He shook his head and smiled. "You're incorrigible."

I tried to curtsey but lost my balance and fell onto the bed, laughing. Bill handed me the cane.

"Behave yourself."

"Guess what happened when I got this darn thing?"

"Do I want to know?"

"Of course you do!" I exclaimed. "I was coming back to the room from PT with this thing stretched across my lap. I must have hit the end of it with my arm because it slipped." I took a breath, hung my head, and quickly added, "I jammed it into the spokes on the wheelchair."

He set down the card he'd opened and looked at me over his glasses, which were resting on the bridge of his nose. "How fast were you going?"

I thought for a minute, trying to decide if I should tell him the truth. Common sense was beginning to seep back into my damaged brain; it just hadn't filtered to my mouth. "I did my first wheelie."

"In other words, you were flying like a bat outta—"

"Thank you for not saying *old*," I interrupted. "And, yes. Yes, I was."

"So, what happened?"

"The maintenance crew was working in the room next to where I locked gears. It took them *five* minutes to get me untangled."

Bill rolled his eyes. "Would you like to get dressed now?"

I looked at the beautiful, peach-colored pantsuit lying on the bed, so feminine with the intricate scrolling on the bodice. The cream-colored, one-inch heels were the perfect choice to wear with this outfit. Another first—a much dreamed about departure from gym shoes.

St. Joseph's Roman Catholic Church is a majestic, Spanish-styled structure. The sanctuary floor is in the shape of a cross with the altar the centerpiece of the gathering space. It's elevated three steps above the main floor. The choir is seated behind the altar. On the wall behind them hangs a simple cross adorned with the risen Lord. The congregation occupies the pews in the main gathering space and the north-side and south-side alcoves.

Bill rolled me to the south side of the sanctuary floor and positioned the wheelchair in the first row of pews closest to the main space.

"I can keep an eye on you from here," he said with a wink. "I gotta get to practice." A quick peck on the cheek and he was gone.

I watched as he disappeared. How grateful I was for his love. The patience he'd shown during my moments of frustration and doubt would cause a lesser man to crumble. The gentle embraces he'd freely given when no words seemed adequate filled my soul with peace and hope. The prayers we shared asking for strength to carry us through this ordeal, and the shouts of joy when another barrier had been broken, were healing glue for my torn spirit.

Silent tears spilled from my eyes this morning and dropped from my cheeks onto the peach-colored jacket, leaving a thin trail of wet.

The church filled to overflowing. It was a day to welcome the faithful, the biannual Christians, those seeking a faith-filled experience, and those who were only there because it was the family thing to do.

I closed my eyes and began to pray.

A sudden lurch of the wheelchair made me realize it wasn't the Holy Spirit moving me. I tried to look over my shoulders to see who was behind me and could see no one. Just as panic seized my throat, I realized a man, a stranger, was moving me partially into the aisle, but just far enough so his family could sit together. He was dressed in a new suit, his hair slicked back and combed wet from a hurried shower. He stunk of aftershave, the kind kids buy as a Christmas gift. He probably used it when he went to the occasional church function: funerals, weddings . . . Easter services.

He never said a word. A sideways glance and a disingenuous smile that quickly disappeared was the only acknowledgement I received from him before he turned his back on me to face his family.

"Good morning," the cantor bellowed cheerfully.

"Good morning," we responded in unison.

"We welcome you on this glorious day. Let's take a moment and say hello to the people sitting nearest you."

Papers rustled as attendees closed their hymnals and greeted the people around them.

There was no one to the side of me, only the aisle. I couldn't twist to see who was behind me. The altar was in front and this man and his family to my left.

I watched as he hugged his wife and, in turn, each of his children. He walked back to his seat, looked at me, and shrugged his shoulders.

"Huh, nobody else here, I see."

He reopened his hymnal and remained standing as the congregation began to recite the opening prayer.

I remained seated, eye-to-belly level with this stranger. I lifted the footrests of the wheelchair with the toes of my cream-colored heels and pursed my lips when I saw the scuff mark left behind.

Somehow, my fingers made it to this man's coat pocket and I gave a tug.

He turned his head partially to the side, looking into his pocket before looking at me.

I placed my hands on the armrests of the wheelchair. This skinny, frail, shadow of a woman with the balance of a marionette gone rogue slowly rose from her seat.

The choir belted out Handel's "Hallelujah" chorus and the congregation chimed in.

"Oh no!" the man shouted above the music as he witnessed my rise from the ashes.

He nervously held his hands in front of me and shook them side to side as though that would signal me to stop. His jittery voice spilled from his lips, commanding, "D-Don't. Don't do that."

His eyes darted around the church, looking for help, an usher, a priest, anyone!

I stood tall that morning, all ninety-eight pounds of me. In a clear voice and with a steady gaze that met his frightened eyes, I softly said, "I am somebody."

CHAPTER TWENTY

MANNERS BE DAMNED!

"Everything in a rehab center is measured," the nurse bemoaned. "Food, water, medicine in, everything expelled . . . including farts, I'm sure," Jackson growled, "are marked and calculated on a chart somewhere."

He circled the room methodically. The nostrils of a dragon-tattoo flared on his wrist from under his long-sleeved shirt when he reached to open the blinds—evidence of biker days gone by.

"There are clipboards at the end of each bed. Papers hanging on every door and volumes on the two of you at the nurse's station," he said. He pointed directly at each of us, one at a time. "My arms are full of files, but do you think I can find one pen?"

Cody and I shrugged our shoulders in sympathy until I let out a honk and she squealed.

He stopped abruptly. "What?"

I pointed at his beard.

"I found it," he said with exuberance. "I knew it was here somewhere."

He began scrawling large, repetitive circles on the top page of the first chart, lines that bore holes into the paper.

"Damn, it's outta ink," he replied through gritted teeth. He pitched the load of papers in his arms onto the end of Cody's bed.

"I'll be back," Jackson said, using his best Arnold Schwarzenegger impression.

When he returned, his hand bulged with pens like a new father passing out cigars after the birth of a child. "This should keep me going until the shift change."

"When's that?" Cody asked.

He looked at his watch. "Twenty-eight minutes from now."

"They told me the party was in here," Bill said as he entered the room.

"Have a pen, sweetie." I grinned.

Bill looked confused by our inside joke but placed his new treasure into his shirt pocket.

"Lost mine," Jackson said, holding one up. "The sleuth sisters found it."

"Oh," Bill said with an approving nod and two thumbs up.

"Hey, I hear y'all are doing something special today," Jackson said.

"I've got a four-hour pass! I'm going home. First time in two months."

"Enjoy every minute of it, honey. You've earned it."

I grinned again. I couldn't wait.

A din of traffic noise filtered through the open doors leading to the pool. It had been a long time since I sprawled on my own bed. It wasn't exactly the way I'd envisioned using two of the four hours on the half-day pass, but I was exhausted from the brief ride home.

"A nap!" I complained.

I tossed off the fleece comforter like a two year old whose playtime had been interrupted and buried my head into the pillow, trying to sweep the sleep away. The pillow and bed felt familiar, smelled familiar, but didn't have that imprint of home anymore. It's not that I didn't recognize them as my own. Instead, I felt like a visitor. I suppose Shakespeare, or Scooby, would have put it this way: a cameo actor on the world's stage waiting to exit . . . stage left.

"You're awake," Bill said cheerfully and plopped on the edge of the bed.

"What time is it?" I asked and rolled towards him. My eyes were still closed. A loose strand of hair curled into the corner of my mouth just as Bill bent to kiss me. I gave a "pffft!" and brushed the hair and his face aside.

He looked stunned.

I gaped in shock, but a smirk began to show on one side of my face. "I'm so sorry."

He feigned hurt. "I thought you liked my kisses."

"I love your kisses. It's the hair . . ."

The ringing phone startled both of us.

"Hello?" Bill said.

"Who is it?" I mouthed.

"Connie," he mouthed back. "Sure. We'll meet you there in fifteen."

"Are we going out to dinner?" I asked, hoping my instinct was right.

"Yep."

"Good. I'm starving!"

I propped myself up on my left side and rolled my feet to the floor. It was an intoxicating experience to be independently mobile again, albeit unsteady. I was eager to try my *new feet* in public without the use of a cane.

The restaurant and parking lot were filled to overflowing. Florida was in the height of snowbird season. Tourists, on the verge of exhaustion created by too many long hours on the road, or suffering from too much Florida sun, or both, lounged on wingback rocking chairs on the restaurant's long porch. Hungry people waited patiently to hear their names called for dinner.

We squeezed past the crowd milling in the general store. Cash registers dinged like slot machines dropping coins as satisfied customers checked out. They held their packages and doggie bags tucked under their arms as they made their way to the exit. I headed upstream from the crowd toward a rack filled with greeting cards.

"I'm going to add our names to the waitlist," Bill said. "You'll be fine here. Don't wander off."

Engrossed in a card, I nodded yes as Bill walked away.

A mother and her two young girls huddled to my

right, giggling over a humorous birthday card. To my left stood a man nearly seven feet tall, shaped like the Pillsbury Doughboy. His ivory white legs extruded from the bulk bursting through his shorts. The waist-band slouched beneath his belly. We looked at each other, smiled, and turned back to reading the cards in our hands.

"Glim, party of three. Glim," crackled the announcement over the loud speaker. I looked around for our neighbor, Connie. She wasn't there yet. Bill was nowhere to be seen, probably in the washroom. The hostess at the far end of the building, surrounded by people, ticked off the names on her list of waiting diners as they stepped forward. The way I saw it, it was up to me to get there before she gave our table away.

I clutched the waist-high counter holding the card rack. My legs were weak from standing too long. I needed to steady my balance before I started walking towards the giant stranger. He glanced in my direction and turned back to the cards. There was no way I could make it around him unless he moved.

I stood close enough to count the hairs in his nose before politely clearing my throat to get his attention. He didn't budge. In fact, he turned his back on me. My words still slurred, so I knew he'd never understand me over the crowd noise.

This man was standing between me and food. I did not think of the appropriate behavior or the repercussions for my actions. My needs and desires were basic.

I'm hungry. The food is there. I'm here. You're in my way.

I looked at that puffy, white skin exploding from those obscenely short shorts, and before I realized it, I'd backhanded him on the butt. THWACK!

The stranger shot straight up and landed two feet away in the middle of an intersecting aisle. His posture was rigid, arms straight at his sides. Only his head moved side to side, eyes round with surprise. I marched past, feeling like a brave little ant in the shadow of an elephant.

"And you know what?" I said with pride the following morning when I retold this story to the occupational therapist. "Mission accomplished."

Paula pulled a chair next to my bed and took my hands in hers. She looked me straight in the eyes. Her gaze was filled with love and sadness, the kind a parent feels for a child who's acted poorly. She sighed.

"Miss Jo Ann, we need to talk about your manners."

CHAPTER TWENTY-ONE

CPR FOR THE SOUL

WHEN I WAS TOLD I had a full-day pass, Bill asked me where I wanted to go. There was no hesitation in my answer. "To the beach!"

I dug my toes deep into the sand dune that separated the parking lot from the strip of powdery white shoreline and the gulf-coast waters beyond. A few steps over the boardwalk and the weight of everyday life slipped to the ground, along with our towels and flip-flops.

Grains of sand and tiny, crushed shell shards snuggled easily between our toes and stuck to the soles of our feet. Feeling was slowly returning to my paralyzed foot. The sensation from the sand felt more like tiny pinpricks than a tickle, and that made my unsteady gait over the sand dune look more like a full-body hiccup.

There were footprints of every size and shape etched into the sand by thousands of beachgoers. The ripple of ruts left behind challenged my weakened legs to climb. The exhilaration of the moment kept me focused on the water's edge. We walked for what seemed to be miles, but in actuality was less than fifty yards at high tide.

Bill held me tightly. He was the only cane I had with me that day. The only one I needed.

"Look!" I pointed with the excitement of a child. The fin of a dolphin broke the smooth surface of the gulf waters. Soon another joined, and another. The last one leapt high into the air in a twirling motion and landed on its side with a resounding splash.

"Wow! That was amazing."

Bill curled his arms around my waist. "Why don't we rest awhile?" he suggested and nodded in the direction of a dry sand mound not too far from the shoreline.

"That sounds good."

He leaned back and propped his long, tan body on the crook of his elbows. I held my legs close to my body and rested my chin on my hands and my elbows on my knees. We smiled as we watched a group of children play dare with the breakers washing to shore.

My stint in rehab had turned into months, and it wasn't over yet. The world as I knew it had become a cocoon of pastel-colored walls and soft lighting. To be lounging on a beach, watching the sun play hide-and-seek with clouds freckling the sky, spanned more freedom of space than I could tolerate. I put my head down and closed my eyes.

"You okay?" Bill asked.

"Yeah. I will be."

"What's going on?"

"I just discovered why children sometimes panic when they're in an unfamiliar place."

"Why?"

"Because, the world is just too big."

⚓

I awakened to the sounds of waves rolling to shore and the squeals of kids as sea foam surrounded their ankles and pulled the sand out from under their feet.

Every breath I took was like a count of CPR for my battered body and soul. Life's energy was slowly returning, all six senses caressed by the forces of nature. So grateful to be alive.

The beach was filled with dots of towels and colorful sun umbrellas. When we first arrived that morning, the air carried a hint of sea salt. Now it hung heavy with sunblock and barbeque.

Bill was smiling down at me with two cold drinks in his hands. He intentionally held them so the ice water trickled down my bare belly.

"Oh, that feels good," I said.

We sat, and sipped, and talked about everything: life, family, the future. Finally, I asked him, "Do you have a special place you're drawn to when you're hurting?"

Bill stroked his chin. "Besides church, I find balance in nature, especially near the ocean, or mountains and woods."

"Me too. That's why I wanted to come here today."

"I know," he said. He slipped his hand under mine and gently held on.

"Did you ever wonder why there's such a pull between

man and the sea?" I asked.

"I don't know." He began to laugh. "The way I look at it, we spent nine months swimming in the womb. There must be a familial sense of unity there somewhere."

He interlocked his fingers behind his head, forming a natural pillow on top of the sand. "Besides that, our bodies are sixty percent water."

"Huh. Imagine that." My index finger traced an infinity sign in the slip of sand between us. The bright sun caused me to squint as I looked toward the water. "When I look at the gulf, I'm struck by the fact that there's as much life under the sea as here on earth. What I can't figure out is why are we looking for aliens in space when they're footsteps, or should I say fin flaps away?"

"When I look at this body of water," Bill said, "I'm awestruck by her beauty."

We slid our sunglasses on and stared at the ribbons of green and blue that stretched as far as the eye could see. Only a thin line of gray separated sea from sky on the horizon.

"She's the perfect analogy for God," I said.

"How do you figure?"

"She's amazing. She's powerful. She's cleansing. She can guide us to other shores. She sustains life."

"And how does God figure into an undertow?" Bill asked.

"That's a terrifying thought," I replied.

Thinking out loud, I slowly surmised, "The senses are totally blocked. We wouldn't know what's up or what's down. When we thrash against the sea, we churn up more sediment . . ."

"What do you do?" he asked, playing devil's advocate.

I thought for a moment before answering, "Surrender."

"Huh, interesting." He was quiet for a moment before he responded, "When you surrender in water, you float."

"Yep."

"So, what you're saying in this metaphor is that when life drags you down, and you can't see your way to a solution, instead of relying on your own resources, which may create more turmoil, you surrender . . . to God. Right?"

"That's exactly what I'm saying. Of course, not everyone believes in God in the same way, but this is what I believe." My voice trailed off as I thought about the stroke; my continuing struggle to find order in everyday living; the days of uncertainty and doubt; and the grueling hours of therapy to relieve the paralysis and weakness.

"One of the lessons I've learned through this whole ordeal is when we battle a devastating attack, God teaches us the true meaning of power, and peace, and inner-strength through surrender."

Bill gingerly applied sunblock to his already tender nose. "Wow. Those are lessons not easily learned, nor always appreciated."

"I can't argue with you about that."

Storm clouds gathered to the north far out to sea.

We watched a lightning strike hit the water. "How can anyone look at the gulf and not feel the presence of God?" I asked.

"I don't know," Bill said and shrugged his shoulders. He stood up and shook the sand from his beach towel. My gaze stayed focused on the horizon.

To the west, the sun's rays hung low in the sky and skipped across the waves like sprites dancing on the tips. This beautiful day would soon be over. It was time to go.

CHAPTER TWENTY-TWO

LAST DAY ON THE MAT

For a stroke survivor, regaining strength cannot be measured in monumental leaps, but rather small, laborious tasks mastered over long periods of time. When the body's been trampled, nothing is instant.

"What you've gained will not last unless you continue to work at it," Nancy said. Her tone was the most serious I'd heard. She had me on my back on the mat, knees bent—slowly pushing the right knee toward my shoulder. "You've got to stay strong and flexible."

"I'll do my best."

"I know you will. I'm on this mat with you, girl."

"Oh, yeah? I don't see any sweat on your forehead."

"That's because I'm southern. I only get dewy."

With my knees still bent and arms flat on the mat, Nancy called the next exercise: "Butt off the ground, raise that right leg, and count to five. Repeat with your left. Let's move it!"

I could feel the blood rushing to my head.

"Hang in there. You've got this!" Nancy yelled while

clapping a cadence for the exercise. Her enthusiasm was contagious. My body's eagerness to keep up with her was not.

It was my last physical therapy workout session at the rehab center. I looked around the room with what surprised me—a bit of nostalgia. I thought about the first time I came in here and how horrified I was when I saw myself for the first time. It's hard to imagine how far I'd come, especially when I still tired so easily.

I was blest to have an outstanding team of therapists, men and women who believed in me and the possible outcome from their amazing training. The best way to describe their team spirit is: never stop trying until there's nothing left to try.

"Here you go, kiddo," Nancy said as she handed me an eight-by-ten envelope.

"What's this?" I asked.

"Open it."

I flipped through the neatly stapled twenty-three pages of illustrated exercises, two per page. Each pose included detailed instructions, suggested number of repetitions, and degree of difficulty boldly printed next to the pictures.

"I want you to do these every night once you're home." Her eyes scanned my skinny frame. "You're strong enough to do fifty reps." She stopped her order in midstream. A faraway look in her eyes and a methodical finger twitch indicated she was recalculating. "In about thirty minutes."

"In my dreams!" I chuckled. "When I was fifteen . . . maybe."

I thought back to my sophomore year and the challenge of completing one hundred squats in five minutes on a double dare. I walked like Frankenstein for a week.

She studied my face and recalculated the numbers. "Okay. Start with twenty and work up to thirty reps," she said emphatically, "in half an hour."

"I can do that."

"Let's go through them one more time to make sure you know them all. I don't want you to hurt yourself by doing them wrong."

I reached for the beach-sized exercise ball that had drifted to the side of the mat. It easily rolled under my shoulders and supported my head and neck on the curve of the sphere. With feet flat and knees bent, the rest of my body either balanced on the ball or cantilevered into midair. My hands rested quietly on my belly, fingers locked. Methodically, to a count of ten, I kicked my left leg out straight—toes pointed, belly muscles tensed. After five reps, I changed legs. With the first kick out on my right, I began to roll to the side.

Nancy's hand braced my shoulder and returned my body to center. "Make sure Bill spots you when you do these." She leaned towards me until her face was even with mine and said firmly, "Every night."

"I will," I said through gritted teeth. My abs began to scream "Enough!" Beads of sweat glistened on my forehead.

"We're almost done," the physical therapist chirped. She sat cross-legged at my side near the edge of the mat. "Do you feel comfortable with what you know?"

"Sure! Now that I've mastered the backstroke on this darn ball, do you have a plate I can balance on the end of my nose?"

"No. But I may be able to find some tape for your mouth." Nancy grinned. I rolled my eyes. The ball threw me to the mat with a thud.

"I'm going to miss you," Nancy said as she helped me up.

PART FIVE

THE SEARCH FOR SELF

CHAPTER TWENTY-THREE

GOOD-BYES ARE NEVER EASY

I SAT IN THE COMMUNITY CENTER longer than usual this morning. The CNAs were quietly arranging spring flowers on the activities table. A snowy picture flickered on the television in the corner of the room. There was no sound. Just a tap-tap-tapping as a resident tried to fix it with the finger-to-screen approach. Most of the patients were already in therapy sessions. Mine ended Wednesday. A few last-minute details, final instructions, and release papers to sign, and I'd be going home ... today.

My hand traced the full-sized figures painted on the center's thirty-foot wall. The mural began at the hallway door to the resident's rooms on one end and continued to the doorway leading to the patio and pond beyond on the other. It was a nice rendering of Florida life with a gulf-view backdrop. The artist, a patient alumnus of the facility himself, used residents as his subjects. Cody was front and center dressed as a beach waitress in shorts and a tank top and posed taking a food order.

I walked down to the offices and said my good-byes to staff. In the past few months, they had become like family. This was a safe haven. Help was around the corner if I got in trouble, didn't feel good, or just needed to talk.

"You're going to be coming in for out-patient therapy," Paula reminded me.

I'd had a chance to watch her baby bump grow over the months. Her time was coming due. As she manipulated the fingers on my affected hand, we'd talk about her dreams for her upcoming, firstborn child.

"You're not getting rid of us that quickly." Paula flashed a motherly smile. "We're here for you, kiddo."

"I've been looking for you," Bill said. "The car's packed and Cody's waiting to say good-bye."

We walked the hall to my room in silence.

"Good-bye, Snort-Face," Cody cried. Tears formed in the corners of her eyes and wetted the pillow beneath. "I'm going to miss you."

"I'm going to miss you, too."

"Promise you'll come see me."

"You know we will," Bill replied.

Cody hugged him tightly. "I'll never forget my beautiful, blue-eyed Bill."

"We'll never forget you either," I sniffled, choking back tears.

"We've got to go now," Bill said quietly.

"Jo Ann, when you came in here, you were a wreck! Now look at you. You're leaving here a new model."

My laughter was laced with sadness. I wanted Cody to be able to do the same. To get out of that damn chair and walk. It had been a long nine years for her with no end in sight.

"Knock, knock!" Dr. Caleb stood in the doorway with arms outstretched.

"Oh, I'm going to miss you!" I cried and hugged her tightly. My arms and legs began to tremble and the room began to whirl. "I think I'm going to faint," I said weakly.

I felt Dr. Caleb hold me closer. Her arms were strong and comforting. A nurse rolled a wheelchair behind me, and they gently sat me back. My face glowed from perspiration. The episode was brief and within a few minutes, I was joking and talking as though nothing had happened.

"Are you feeling better?" the doctor asked.

"Yeah." I nodded.

"Thank you for everything," Bill said and rolled me toward the side entrance door.

The hallway's lighting was dim. The illusion became a sixty-foot tunnel of beige ceiling, floor, walls, and trim. A small, door-paneled window, inlaid with chicken-wire screening, streamed a channel of light down the tile floor like a luminescent carpet ending at my feet.

It frightened me.

Is this the last scene I'll see before I die? I mused. *Is this what they mean by going toward the light? Did God confuse me with another patient? Was this whole traumatic event the wait between life and death?*

I snapped back to reality when I caught a glimpse of Cara, the day nurse, in Jordan's room as we wheeled by. She was bent over his bed shaving him with a blade. She'd done it the same way every day for the past twelve years. He was a paraplegic and blind, but he could hear and—he could scream. It was his only form of vocalization. Depending on his needs, his screams could be abrupt or shrill or if he was singing with Cara, long. The light from the window in his room haloed Cara's golden-blond hair and bathed his face in radiance. I felt honored and a little embarrassed to have witnessed this tender and private moment.

Mrs. Hartwell's groans filled the air from a darkened room along the hallway. She called out to her dead husband, "Charles, is that you?" This was a phrase repeated every time someone walked past her door.

Maybe that light was meant for her, I thought. *Maybe it's Charles knocking at the side entrance. DO NOT OPEN THAT DOOR!* my mind screamed as a CNA let Mr. Bailey in. The dapper old man had been sitting in the parking lot enjoying his morning cigar, unaware that the door locked behind him. Mr. Bailey was in his sixties, always nicely dressed, always pleasant, always disappearing. He never wandered far. He just never thought to tell anyone where he was going.

Everyone knew where to find Mr. Bailey on bath day, though. He'd be first in line for the showers. Sometimes, he'd get his days confused. First order of business for the CNAs was to lift the curtain and check for Mr. Bailey's bare legs when it was women's shower day—not that he was interested in seeing something he shouldn't; he just liked to look his best, and that began with a shower.

Mr. Bailey tipped his hat as we passed. I smiled and extended my hand to him.

"Good-bye, my dear lady."

"Good-bye, Mr. Bailey."

We rolled past the library. Even though it was empty, I could hear the echo of Dr. Finkle telling me, "Remember . . . you are still you."

Somehow, I felt abandoned by the very people who had taken such good care of me. I felt anger toward the little creatures I call THEY who decide a person's fate from a distance based on HMOs, PPOs POSs, and bottom-line economics.

I wanted to leave through the front double doors with a large bouquet of flowers on my lap. I wanted doctors and therapists, nurses, and administrators standing along the corridor, applauding as I passed by.

Come on, people! If the wait staff in a restaurant can drop everything to sing a silly rendition of "Happy Birthday," you *can* do this. This had been a life-altering event and I SURVIVED! YAHOO!!!

Nobody asked me what I wanted or how I felt about the transition to home. THEY, those little creatures, said it was time to go.

I wasn't ready.

CHAPTER TWENTY-FOUR

REPELLED BY THE FAMILIAR

TODAY WAS MY FIRST full day at home. I kept avoiding Bill. I didn't want him to know how confused and depressed I felt. This wasn't the reaction I expected from my homecoming, and I'm sure it was not the one he anticipated either.

I never felt this way when I had a half-day pass. It was wonderful to be surrounded by our personal belongings; to watch the dog's silly antics for those few precious hours; and to languish on our deck, enjoying the warm air and gulf breezes. These were cherished, quiet moments alone with my husband. No pressures. No thoughts of life before the stroke or after, just grateful for life.

Today, pure emotional sludge percolated from my toes to my brain, choking out all sensibilities. *Why do I feel like this? Where is this anger coming from? I feel so alone, so useless.*

Bill cautiously peeked into the darkened den. "I'm going to the store. Do you need anything?"

"I'm almost out of soda," I mumbled from under the blanket, my face buried toward the back of the couch.

"You got it."

"And tissues."

"Okay." He nodded and blew me a kiss.

I blew my nose.

It's funny how you get used to certain sounds like the squeak of the garage door when it drops the last three inches to the concrete below. I listened to the hum of the car's engine until I could hear it no more. This was the first time in over three months I was alone, completely alone. Not a call button in sight, no one in the hall pushing a pill cart.

I stood in the passageway behind the living room couch and looked out the window towards the woods. It was easy to do. New house . . . no curtains. The night before the stroke, I'd completed a panel of sheers for one of the two sliding doors leading to the pool. It looked nice, even though it wasn't hemmed or pinned. The curtain for the other door's window was still a piece of material neatly folded and tucked in a corner out of sight.

My good hand mindlessly massaged the palm of the partially paralyzed, and still swollen, one. Feeling and movement were slowly returning . . . very slowly. With great difficulty, I could touch the tip of my thumb to the tips of each finger. The motions were awkward and bumbling. Threading a needle and creating a succession of uniform stitches was out of the question for now.

I sighed as I sat at the dining room table, gazing at the four-by-eight-foot photograph hanging on the wall. It was a magnificent sunset shot taken at our favorite beach in the Pacific Northwest; so many happy memories were attached to Sunset Beach, my childhood playground. Ironically, that picture may have documented my last trail hike. I didn't know if I would ever climb on rocks, or explore tide pools, or slide over driftwood logs again. The goal today is walking.

I wandered from room to room. So many things I'd taken for granted. So many treasures tucked into "someday-I'll-get-to-this" drawers: trinkets and jewelry; designer paper; sample-size jars of paint; even slides from all over the world waited to be archived. Many earmarked for gifts. Hah! Not now.

I wondered . . . will I ever use my hands in a creative way again? Hold a camera? Change lenses? Paint an intricate pattern? Do needlework?

I hung my head and sobbed. *I can't hold a full glass of water without dropping it! The family applauds when I finish a meal and my fork is still in my hand.*

Bill and I had dreamt about this move for years; our retirement nest away from brutally cold Chicago winters. This was to be our time to enjoy life and the simple pleasures. Now, nothing was simple. Brushing my teeth was a full morning ritual. The toilet seat was equipped with handrails. I couldn't shower unless I sat on a chair.

I collapsed onto the couch in the den, again feeling

the cool damp from tears already wept as I buried my head into the pillow. I didn't want to see anybody. I didn't want to talk to anybody. I just wanted to dissolve into the cushions.

I spent four days in self-appointed hell isolated in that twelve-by-fourteen-foot room. A million questions darted through my mind with barbs aimed at my very soul. *Why didn't I die? Why am I still here? I have nothing left to offer. Bill doesn't deserve to be saddled with an invalid wife. It's not fair! How am I supposed to live like this? How are* we *supposed to live like this?*

Uncontrollable sobs strangled my throat. I was drowning in grief and sorrow. What little sleep I got was swaddled in exhaustion, and then . . . all was quiet the morning of the fifth day.

Not one tear left in those red, swollen eyes. Not one sob formed in my quiver-free lungs. I inhaled like someone starving for oxygen. My head throbbed, but not one negative thought bounced through the twisted trough of my mind. The recesses purged of all negativity.

A ladder of morning light streamed through the partially closed blinds and cast a broad beam over the puffs of used tissues piled next to the couch. My mother's voice echoed in my mind, repeating the last words of wisdom she shared with me before she died.

"Don't. Ever. Quit."

CHAPTER TWENTY-FIVE

LIE VERY, VERY STILL

I FLIPPED THE DOG-EARED pages of a two-year-old magazine I'd found on a rack next to the check-in window at the diagnostic center. A few more hours, one final test, and I'd be medically released.

Free. Free at last! No more physical therapy. No more doctors' appointments. No more tests!

My therapist's parting words rose above the clamor of my happy thoughts like a soloist in a church choir. "Keep up with physical therapy on your own *every* day," she vocalized with gusto. "Otherwise, you'll lose everything you've gained so far."

To that, the chorus that lives in my mind harmonized, "Oooooooh, lose it...lose it. Going, going, gone. Bye-bye!"

I snorted with a breath of contempt but knew in the end I'd do it. I was not about to risk forfeiting what I'd achieved.

"Mrs. Glim?" the technician trumpeted in a high, whiny voice. His tall, thin body eclipsed the doorway.

Odd thing was, his torso faced me, but his feet were planted in the opposite direction, ready to walk the long corridor. It was a position I don't think a dancer from the Bolshoi ballet could have duplicated.

I nodded and fumbled with the strap on my purse. Bill gathered my other belongings, and we walked behind the tech like an obedient pair of ducklings.

The MRI machine was the main event in the darkened room. A blackout shade over the only window on the outside wall allowed splinters of bright light to filter in as a pulsing, one-inch orb around the opening.

Oversized prints of Florida landscapes adorned the deep-colored walls. One crème-colored sofa, a desk and chair, and a hook for clothing and personal items completed the room's sparse decor.

The machine, tethered with electrical and computer wires, looked like a cylindrical space capsule turned on its side. At the far end, where a booster rocket would normally be, was a gaping hole, large enough to accept a man lying prone. A dark red, leather mattress jutted into the room. To my weakened eyes, it resembled a metal prototype of the Rolling Stones' *Forty Licks* album cover.

"I want you to lie here," the tech said as he slapped the taut, red leather platform. His hand left a momentary imprint in the still-drying antiseptic wash.

"It's very important that you lie very, very still," the tech whispered as though talking too loudly would wake the beast within the machine. "This is a *very* sophisticated piece of equipment." I waited for him to cross himself and was relieved when he didn't. "It takes pictures of your body in very thin, slice form."

My eyes darted from one manufacturer's label inside the tube to another. Fortunately, none said *deli*.

"These slices are studied individually. They may also be overlaid to give the doctor a *very* detailed look at the area of your body we're going to study today."

"Hmmm." I responded. "Okay."

"And what area will we study today?" he asked condescendingly as he slowly rolled me into the capsule.

"Don't you know?" My eyes widened with surprise. I was totally enclosed in the capsule by now, my nose three inches from the interior wall of the unit.

"Yes, Mrs. Glim, we know. We just want to make sure you know," he said and wiggled my big toe.

Oh, I wanted to say my foot, but before my thalamus-inflicted mind could spurt out foot, my better self convinced me that I really didn't want to spend any more time in rehab.

"My brain," I dutifully responded.

"*Very* good."

He snuggled a blanket around my legs. The chill in the room reminded me of a cool autumn morning in the Midwest. I appreciated the added warmth.

"The machine's going to make a noise similar to a jack hammer. This will protect your ears from the noise," he said and slipped cushioned headphones over my ears. He handed me a substantially large, round object attached to a wire.

Between being in an enclosed space, the reverberation of my voice in that area, and the microphone in my hand, I felt like I was back at the radio station doing voice-overs.

"If you listen to the music, it'll help pass the time. So, just relax and try not to move."

"Okay," I said. Then an odd silence filled the room. I realized I was alone. "Hey," I called. There was no response. The machine was beginning to whirr and thunk. "Hey," I said again, this time a little louder. Still nothing. "What am I supposed to do with this microphone?" I yelled. "Is this a part of the test?"

I listened but didn't hear anything. *Did he tell me but I forgot? Did he forget to tell me? All this money for this test and we may have to do it again?*

I sighed and pulled the cord down tightly so the foam ball rested in the crook of my fingers, then brought the microphone to my lips. It was hard to form notes with my damaged vocal cords, but if they expected a medical version of karaoke, I'd give it my best, albeit a little loud and a lot off key.

"Our house . . . is a very, very, very fine house . . . with two cats in the yard . . ."

One of my favorite groups, Crosby, Stills, and Nash before Young. *Love this song.* I took a deep breath and was ready to belt it out when I felt a hand shake my knee.

"Mrs. Glim!" The voice shouted in high C. "You must remain perfectly still during this test."

"Then why did you give me a microphone?"

"That's not a mic," the tech said. His words spilled out between bouts of laughter. "It's the call button in case you need me."

⌘

Bill waited for the caller to identify himself before answering the phone.

"Do you mind if I put you on speaker phone so we can both hear what you have to say?"

He placed the phone on the coffee table between our chairs. "It's the doctor's office, sweetie, with the MRI results."

"Hello! We're both here," I replied.

"Well, I have good news and I have even better news. We'll start with the good. As you know, most strokes are caused by a clot that interrupts the flow of blood to the brain. Yours was caused by a tear in a vessel. Even though the stroke occurred in a minor vein, it caused significant injury. Blood being like water, it seeks the path of least resistance. So, before the bleeding stopped, the pressure pushed against the creases of the brain and caused substantial damage. However, it seeped slowly enough so as not to tear any vital pathways and cause permanent harm."

"I knew there was a reason I'm not good at math. The wires aren't connected."

Bill just shook his head. "You have more news, Doctor?"

"I have great news," Dr. Caleb said. "There's no sign

of another aneurysm. There are no tumors. There's no blood clot. As a matter of fact," she said cheerfully, "there's nothing there."

I looked at Bill through squinted eyes.

He just grinned and said, "Thank you, Doctor, for verifying what we already knew."

CHAPTER TWENTY-SIX

THINK ABOUT IT

I CAUGHT MY REFLECTION in the floor-to-ceiling mirrors across the room at the rehab center's therapy area. I was amazed how far I'd come since the first time I glimpsed my crumpled form slumped in a wheelchair three months ago. A slight smile curled my lip, and I shamelessly winked at myself. *You go, girl* was the rallying cry for my day. I stood up with no assistance and stretched my arms out straight from my sides. With every movement my mind shouted, *Thank you, God!*

I walked toward Nancy. It was a nice surprise to see she was the outpatient therapist for the day. This was a rotated position. You never knew who you were going to get. We were both wearing ear-to-ear grins, but not for the same reason.

"What I'm holding in my hand is just for you!" she announced.

I had no idea what she was talking about, and it showed on my face.

She placed a pile of official-looking papers on the table in front of me.

"I caught wind of a new program they're setting up at the hospital. There's only a handful of patients who could possibly do this because of what y'all have been through. You'd be a perfect match for the team."

"Perfect for what?" I glanced at my right hand, the one that had been so severely damaged by the stroke. Slowly, the swelling was going down, but the fingers still had a will of their own.

Nancy saw my reaction and quietly said, "Perfect for helping others struggling with what you experienced." She took a deep breath.

"They're starting a peer counseling program to help stroke survivors and their families understand what it's like from the point of view of the survivor. You will be a voice for those who cannot speak for themselves."

She rested her elbows on the table and waited for a response from me. It was slow coming.

"So. Whadaya think?"

"I don't know what to think." I flipped through the papers before answering.

"Anybody who suffers a brain attack never fully returns to what society considers normal. Suffering a stroke is a metamorphic catastrophe—psychologically, emotionally . . ."

"Physically," Nancy added.

"And spiritually."

"I know," Nancy said quietly. "I see patients every day who fight to regain what they've lost. A stroke occurs with such dramatic and devastating results. In the beginning, we have no way of telling if a patient will return to a functioning life. Because it takes so much time and effort, some of them just give up."

"And sometimes," I added, "we're told we'll never be able to do something and believe it, rather than continuing to try." Sadness washed over me. "How do I encourage others to set personal goals? To go for it, even if they've been told they may never do it again? Whatever it is?"

"That's one of the reasons the hospital's setting up a peer counseling program," Nancy explained, "to help everyone realize they're not alone during the healing process, that much of what they think and feel is universal, and that there is hope."

My mind flashed back to my own experience. "It takes a long time to realize and process everything that's happened. My recovery was fairly quick. Some patients, depending on the severity of their stroke, may never recover much function. I would never want to offer them false hope."

"From what I read in your files, your stroke should have been fatal."

I nodded. "That's true."

"This is exactly what the families of stroke survivors need to hear. We all feel you could offer a perspective to patients and their loved ones that none of us can because you experienced it, lived through it, and by the grace of God and a miraculous recovery, you have the opportunity to share that message with others."

"Do you think because I'm no longer wheelchair bound or noticeably physically impaired, patients will question if I truly understand what they're facing? Have I healed so well they'll think I don't remember?"

I heard a click of heels on the tile floor coming our way. "You may have to wait until you meet with a patient to find the answer to that. Besides, you'll go through intensive training with the medical and therapy staff." I could smell Dr. Caleb's perfume before I felt her hand on my shoulder. Her presence always lifted my spirit.

"Whatever you'd say would help keep the survivor's demons at bay. It might even save wear and tear on our fire doors." She laughed and gave me a wink.

An audible gasp blew past my lips. "How did you know about that?"

"We all knew," Nancy said, joining in the laughter.

"So, are you going to do it?" Dr. Caleb asked.

"Do you think I should?"

"I was the first to recommend you."

"What if I say the wrong thing? I don't want to leave people with misinformation, and I certainly don't want to depress them."

I felt like my soul had been laid bare in the blazing sun, an object for all to see and devour with a critic's knife. Those who did not understand were free to rip it apart and spit the partially chewed pieces back at my feet. Was I willing to share so intimately? Could my story actually help others? The stroke had pulled me into another dimension in minutes, and just as quickly, within months, I physically returned to an active life. Shredded around the edges, but a lot more grateful and hyper-aware of how quickly our personal journey can push us over a cliff.

"There may always be something to remind you of your limitations," Nancy said.

"And that's not a bad thing," Dr. Caleb added.

My thoughts turned to Margi, the night nurse who nearly died in a car accident a few years back. Her willingness to let me feel the indentation in her skull, a residual from flying through the windshield, and the fact that she had not gone to nursing school until after the accident inspired me to do my best while I was in rehab.

I finally understood what Nancy and Dr. Caleb were trying to say.

I grabbed their hands, took a deep breath, and groaned. "Before I talk myself out of doing this, I'm telling you . . . I'll do it."

CHAPTER TWENTY-SEVEN

WHY NOW?

THERE WAS NOT A SOUND in the house. No whir or clink or hum, only the distant tick-tock of the pendulum on the cuckoo clock at the far end of the living room. I woke up lying on my back, hands crossed upon my chest, and my head gently cradled on the pillow.

There was no particular noise that startled me. In fact, it was more the lack of sound, a deafening silence, that interrupted my rest. If I turned my head to look at the alarm, I could see it was 4:00 a.m. Every night the same time, and not because the clock is broken. I've checked.

The slowly turning bedroom fan threw abstract shadows across the ceiling. Every morning, I saw the same benign vision, but in my sleep-altered state, it was a flurry of charging minions from the grim reaper. Angels of death reaching toward me, too far to touch flesh, yet close enough to blow kisses that glance across my cheeks like stones skipped in a lake.

"What the hay!" I rubbed the sleep from my eyes.

"You better be gone," I growled and rolled to my side. *What next, flying monkeys? It's no wonder I feel like death is a heartbeat away.*

"Oh yeah?" Bill shouted. "Garuphical."

I pressed my face into the pillow to stifle a laugh. Bill swears he doesn't talk in his sleep or snore. *One day, I'm gonna record his more memorable sounds and grunts and one-word retorts. Too tired right now.*

My leg felt more numb than usual. I drew circles under the covers with my ankles, toes rolling in unison from left to right. Sometimes, the extra motion improved circulation and made the stroke-affected leg feel more comfortable. Tonight the movement caused the sheets to pull over Bill's feet and, with a few unrefined words, he turned to his other side. I held my breath, hoping I didn't wake him.

How long will this early morning ritual plague me? So far, it's been every night since I came home. Asleep one moment, awake the next. The good news is I'm still a part of this world. I'm alive. Really alive! Although, sometimes, I believe this is a flash of legacy before my life on earth is ultimately over.

"STOP IT!" I hiss out loud.

"Whaaat?" Bill mumbled.

"Go back to sleep, honey. It's just gas."

"Oh!" He scrunched his face and flapped the sheets.

"Yours, not mine," I replied.

He stopped flapping.

I closed my eyes and tried not to laugh, or cry. My head ached from fighting against the feelings of dread.

I wish I could turn on the television. The mindless chatter of rerun news usually bores me back to sleep, but I don't want to wake Bill.

I quietly lay there waiting for dawn, too sleepy to settle into my chair in the den, too conscious to ignore the thoughts pushing into my mind with the force of a tsunami.

Predawn light seeped through our bedroom window, signaling the hour before sunrise. I said my morning prayers and reminded myself that before the stroke, I was self-reliant, independent, and strong. Before the event, I had an army-of-one attitude.

Not anymore, and that's okay. Trauma changes attitude, at least it changed mine. It's trauma, not drama that makes us stronger and puts life squarely in the proper perspective. The small, day-to-day issues were no longer important. Life was now measured in gratitude.

I was grateful for the independence I gained every day. I no longer physically hovered between life and death. Now, it was the mental wrangling with doubts and fears about things that may never happen that kept me wounded. Nothing in life is certain or guaranteed, but somehow I had to relearn to take it on faith that I would awaken to enjoy another day. Enjoy it to the fullest.

Two things are for certain: 1) It's not important if the world is made of gold. ... The question we need to contemplate is: Are we?; and 2) This experience was teaching me that I am not in a hurry to transition to the afterlife, but when the time comes, I no longer fear it.

The sun shone brightly in our bedroom.

"Good morning, sweetheart," Bill said and gave me a smooch.

"Mornin'," I yawned.

Bill rolled out of bed. I pulled the covers over my head.

CHAPTER TWENTY-EIGHT

EARLY MORNING VISITOR

IT WAS FOUR IN the morning again. The bed and I were drenched in sweat. My body trembled, not from chills but emotion. I took a couple of slow breaths and ticked off a mental list of possibilities. Hot flash? No. Stroke? Possibly. Nightmare . . . again? Probably.

Slowly, I flexed my hands, and in a voice barely audible so as not to wake Bill, I sang the alphabet: "A . . . B . . . C . . . D." A sigh of relief calmed me as the letters formed properly on my lips. This was not another stroke, although I feared another one was imminent. I cursed the thought and wondered if it was my destiny to spend the rest of my life waiting.

These nightmares were monstrous intrusions brought on by indiscriminate thieves, namely: anger, fear, and projection. Damn these demons! They pounded at the door of my senses and slithered unnoticed alongside conscious thought. Depression and resignation followed and quietly closed my mind, standing guard over my mouth so I wouldn't cry out for help.

My recollections drifted to a surgery I'd had thirty years ago. That particular night, I'd twisted my body into an impossible position. One leg caught in the side rail of the hospital bed, tubing laced through my fingers like the beginning knot on a macraméd plant hanger. Pressure on the creased, flexible hose strangled the dripline and set off every alarm in the room.

"Miss Jo Ann, are you all right?" the nurse shouted in my ear. She gave me three knuckles to the breastbone.

"Ow! NO," I said and slapped at her arm.

"Oh, sorry," she said and pulled away. She straightened my body and untangled the mash of tubing caught in my hand.

"What on earth happened in here?"

"I don't know. I had a horrible dream!"

"Do you remember it?"

I wish I could erase the scene. "I was on a rickety, old school bus filled with children. The driver was a talking elephant. He said he wasn't feeling good, and then his body just kept getting bigger and bigger until he had all of us pinned to our seats. And then he exploded, BA-LOOSH! There was blood everywhere!"

I began to sob, "I-I can't find the kids."

The nurse burrowed her butt into the well-worn cushion of the visitor's chair and held my hand in hers.

"Honey, a part of this may be the cocktail of drugs we've been feeding you, but I believe it's also a part of the healing process."

She took a butterscotch from her pocket and buried it into her cheek like a ballplayer chucking a wedge of snuff. I could hear her teeth click on the hard candy as she gathered her thoughts.

"When the mind and body are trying to come to terms with a traumatic assault like surgery or stroke or accident, it may appear as some crazy-ass nightmare. It's normal. You're okay. In time, it'll stop."

She was right.

Thirty years later, though, it was happening again; same scenario, different reason, but this time, I had no recollection of any dreams, just an overwhelming feeling of doom. This time, it began months after the actual event. Every morning at four o'clock sharp, the same soaking, the same feeling of terror and abandonment, the same echoes of *why?*

I wanted to curl into a fetal position and rock this misery away. I wanted to hear my mother's soothing voice tell me it was going to be okay. I wanted to be back in that state of calm I felt in the hospital after the event first happened and I thought I was going to die. I wanted to feel the presence of God.

A shimmer of pale light passed the door to our darkened bedroom, the neighbor's car pulling out of their driveway. I waited for the quick toot of the horn. Their way of saying "I love you" before leaving for work. I often wondered why they didn't just say it like the rest of us married folk instead of waking everybody in the neighborhood with that toot.

What the blazes time is it anyway? I sighed and rolled to the side of the bed. *Might as well get up and pee.*

That's when I heard her voice.

"It's going to be okay, sunshine."

"Mom?"

"Uh-huh. In the flesh. Well, not really, but I'm here nonetheless."

"You realize you've been dead sixty years, don't you?"

"Yeah. You realize you didn't have to bury me with my shoes on, right?"

"I thought you wanted to look proper when you met Jesus."

"Jeez, you could have put socks on my feet and tucked the shoes in the bottom of the casket. I could have changed later. Besides, I wanted to be buried in my wedding dress."

"I asked. The funeral director told Grandma it didn't fit. Your arms were too big."

"Well, they'd fit now." I could hear the smile in her voice.

"Why are you here?"

"Do you want me to leave?"

"No! I want you to stay forever. We have so much catching up to do."

"We'll have an eternity to catch up later."

"Then why are you here?"

"You asked for my help. But my time is limited, so talk!"

"I'm having trouble with hideous nightmares."

"Oh, honey, it's just your brain and body having a conversation, actually more like an argument."

"Why now? It's been months since the stroke."

"Their top priority in life is to keep you safe. In this instance, they didn't. Now that they know you're on the road to recovery, they're reviewing what went wrong. When they figure out the details, the nightmares will stop."

"What do I do in the meantime?"

"Count your blessings."

"What?"

"Right now, you're stuck in a cesspool of doubt, and fear, and anger. You can't just will that away. When you stop doing something, it creates a void. Voids demand to be filled. That's why so many people go back to bad habits. They don't think to fill the void."

"Fill it with what?"

"The secret, sweetheart, is to replace it with something positive, so . . . Count. Your. Blessings."

"Besides the litany of things I say all the time, what else do I say?"

"I don't want you to say anything. I want you to think. Think of each person who's helped you throughout this ordeal."

"I do."

"You're not hearing me. Think about all the people, for instance, the housekeeper who quietly cleaned up the mess you made when you accidently spilled that full plate of food onto the floor. She's the one who walked all the way back to the kitchen to get you a new, hot tray of food. Did you know that was her first day back to work after knee surgery?"

"No."

"Think about the therapists who drove to the garden center on their lunch hour and bought potting soil and clay pots and plants, with their own money, so you could work your hands with something you love. They did that to help you heal and make you happy.

These are your shadow angels. They went beyond ordinary care. Remember them and all the others, including family and friends and medical staff. People, even strangers, love you dearly. There's nothing they wouldn't do to help."

"You make ordinary folk sound like superheroes."

"That's exactly what we all can be.

Believe in the goodness of man. It's how God planned for us to live. Our superpower is healing each other through acts of love, and in the end there's only three questions you'll be asked: Did you love others unconditionally? Did you seek wisdom and truth? Did you use your talents and gifts to help others?"

"Mom?"

"Hmmmmm?"

"We used to spend hours talking about everything. I miss it. Even after you died, I heard your voice guide me. I relied on it. And then, one day it was gone. I can tell you exactly when you stopped giving me advice. I was fifty-one years, seven months, and eleven days old. Why did you stop?"

"That's the same age, to the hour, I was when I died."

A look of confusion wrinkled my face.

"From that moment on, you were older than me and would quickly become wiser. Everything I shared with you while you were a child and I still walked the earth, even the things I shared with you when you were an adult and I spoke them to you in conscience, are all stored in your heart. There's nothing more I could offer you."

A kernel of peace blossomed and spread throughout my body as this truth settled in. I felt safe and loved like I did when my mother used to tuck me into bed at night. I felt an all-consuming joy beyond any I've experienced before or since. It was a love that looked beyond my failings and accepted me, just as I am.

"Mom?"

No response.

"Mom?"

Even though she was gone, again, so was the longing for her to be my advocate, my voice, my stanchion in a storm. I knew I would still miss her terribly, but I also knew one day we'd be reunited. One day.

CHAPTER TWENTY-NINE

THE TREK TO ELSEWHERE

ANOTHER HALF HOUR AND we'd see Cody for the first time since she'd moved from the center. The move was a good thing for her. The new facility was closer to her family, but it meant a forty-mile drive for all her old friends.

I pulled the latest copy of *Better Homes and Gardens* out of the gift bag we had for her in the back seat of the car. Even with us going seventy miles an hour, it surprised me to see traffic zipping by so quickly. This was the first highway road trip since the stroke, and my senses were still set to wheelchair speed.

The large, ornate bag overflowed with homemade chocolate chip cookies, body lotion, peach tea, a new beach towel, and tickets to Disney World. The latter was a surprise for Cody. A group of ambulatory patients were scheduled to go to the theme park at Christmastime. We were invited as Cody's guests. We couldn't wait to see her expression when the charge nurse told her we'd been approved.

I flipped pages, looking for a particular article, as Bill pitched coins into the tollbooth's basket.

"Listen to this," I said, clearing my throat before I read. "Gary Legwold, a columnist for the magazine, wrote an article about strokes this month: 'According to statistics, if four people suffer from a hemorrhagic stroke, two will die immediately, the third will die soon after or be severely disabled, and only the fourth will recover with no guarantee as to the quality of their life.'"

"That's almost word for word what Margi told you in rehab."

I nodded my head slowly as I recalled that midnight conversation.

"By the grace of God," I voiced quietly with a slight smile brushing my lips.

"...love from family and friends and the power of prayer," Bill added and winked.

"Dedicated professionals" was my response. By now, Bill and I were both grinning.

This litany was one we repeated often as an informal prayer of thankfulness.

"...and a never-give-up attitude!" he shouted with such fervor I expected to see the Lone Ranger and Tonto ride out of sight.

"I'm making my way back to normal! YEAH!" My hands waved freely in the air as the "William Tell Overture" gained volume in my head.

Cody's new campus was beautiful. We wended our way down a garden path to the fourth building on the left in the enormous multi-unit complex.

"Patient's name?" the receptionist asked while covering

the mouthpiece on her phone. We could hear the unseen caller chatting away. The woman behind the desk pointed toward a short corridor, flipped her hand to indicate another, held up three fingers, and deftly raised her whole arm skyward. Bill answered with a serious pucker and two thumbs up.

The building's newly decorated hallways were lined with patients sitting in wheelchairs. Some slept with their heads resting on their knees. Others cried out the names of loved ones. A few stared straight ahead, unaware of their surroundings.

My cheeks glistened with the moist after-trails of fallen tears. I grabbed Bill's hand as a wave of nausea swept over my body. My hand shook uncontrollably.

"This could have been me in one of these rooms."

"I know," Bill answered. His arm firmly embraced my shoulder.

"Why in God's name was I spared?"

"Honey, I know you're thinking about that forty-nine-year-old medical rep with the four kids and the astronomical mortgage who died unexpectedly last week. The receptionist at the doctor's office should have never told you."

"I understand her shock and pain. He was her friend. But why would she share that story with me when I had just come so close to death myself?"

"Don't allow yourself to be devoured by guilt because you're alive and functioning and someone else isn't. It shouldn't come as a surprise to anyone that we all have an expiration date."

"That's not what's eating me up."

"What then?"

"How do I live with the guilt I feel for not feeling guilty?"

Bill wrapped me in his arms. "You know what? You're right where you're supposed to be."

I realized at that moment what little control each of us has over our destiny. It was also a relief to know that I am not in charge of scheduling. Even though Bill and I worked hard for thirty years, saved and planned to retire early and live where it was warm all year long, nothing prepared us for a major catastrophe like this.

Each of the sweet souls we met today had plans and dreams of their own, too. Separated from family (no matter how nice the facility) is not on any of our wish lists, but rest assured it could and may happen to any one of us.

Society, with our permission, has inundated us with the notion that we're self-sufficient, a master of our own ship, capable of doing it all. Sometimes, life is served to us as a piece of humble pie heaped with self-pride. We are not always the one qualified to offer comfort. Sometimes, we are the one in need.

That's one big piece of pie. I stared at the beauty of Tampa Bay as we headed home.

─◦◦◦─

Bill and I snuggled on the couch that evening, watching an early evening game show. Visions of Cody's new, resident/neighbors floated through my mind. It brought back memories of living in the facility for three months, not knowing if I'd ever be well enough to go home. At that time, the facility seemed more like where I should be—more secure, more comfortable, and structured to fit my needs. Medical help just a call button away.

How different it is living with my sweet hubby again. I wanted this more than anything. I dreamed of resuming our life right where we had left it. But that wasn't our reality. My strength and coordination were far from perfect. Balance mimicked walking a ship's deck during rough seas. I couldn't figure out simple processes like the button sequence to activate the microwave to make a bag of popcorn. I still needed help cutting the meat on my plate. Writing with a pen or pencil looked like scribbles from a three year old. I couldn't shuffle cards without playing 52-pickup, which happened daily, thanks to family and friends who pushed me to improve my dexterity. Dressing became a two-hour ordeal, which led to a four-hour nap.

Everything I did was mentally and physically exhausting. Appointments became planned events. Each activity took thought. If coordinated during a Teflon moment, the thought process in my injured brain tended to quickly slide back into cyberspace, which meant the appointment would be missed.

Most of the time, we found the humor in the "new me." Most of the time, I woke up with a heart grateful for the new day. Most of the time, I joyfully faced any challenge that came our way. Most of the time...

Some days, like today, I had difficulty thinking of

my husband burdened with me for the rest of his life. There were still no guarantees as to how far I could go to return to a life with no restrictions. I struggled with this thought while in rehab, partially because many professional consults began with an inventory of what I may never be able to do again. My heroes were the enthusiastic team of physical therapists who basically responded to that attitude with "We'll see about that!"

As wonderful as it was to see Cody today, the visit placed those negative thoughts front and center in my mind again.

I curled closer to Bill. I could feel his chest rise and fall with every breath he took. The slips of spent air tickled the nape of my neck. It was as comforting to me as when a mother rocks her child to sleep.

This good man deserves so much better than this. He deserves to have a life and not be strapped to an invalid. He deserves to follow his dreams, our dreams, without me holding him back.

Grief filled my heart with sadness as I thought of us parting ways. He's my life! My rock.

I struggled with the notion of him caring for me daily, even though he never complained. He never looked at me in any way but lovingly. He never asked for anything in return. Everyone said what a remarkable recovery I was making. What if it hadn't been so remarkable?

"You look lost in thought," Bill said, running his fingers through my hair.

My chin quivered and I quickly looked away.

"What did I do wrong?" Bill asked.

"Nothing!" I cupped my hands around his face and looked him in the eyes. "Nothing. Oh my gosh, you could not be more perfect."

"What then?"

"I just can't stop thinking about what our lives would be like if circumstances had turned out differently. What if I were still bedridden? Unable to move? How could I possibly expect you to still honor our marriage vows? You deserve happiness. You deserve more."

A look of pain clouded his face. "I would never leave you," he said. His weary voice cracked with hurt.

"I know you wouldn't want to, but you've only one life . . ."

I had no other gift to give him. Even a used tissue could offer a dry corner for a sniffle. I felt depleted as a human being. I had nothing. Giving him his freedom was the purest offering I could make.

"Would you leave me if I had a stroke?" he asked.

"Never!"

That he would even ask shocked me. We were a team. We were on this journey called life together, through it all, good and bad. It was at that moment I realized the true gift we had to offer each other. It wasn't being Rambo-ish and strong at all times. It was to allow the person who was well the freedom to love unconditionally the one ailing while they were at their weakest. Without realizing it, I had taken this loving, selfless gift of my husband's and stomped all over it.

I hid my face in shame and cried.

Bill kissed my tears and quietly responded, "You have my answer. End of discussion."

PART SIX

TRANSITIONS TO A NEW NORMAL

CHAPTER THIRTY

THE GIFT

FIFTEEN MINUTES BEFORE SUNDAY services begin, the church sanctuary is quiet. A handful of the faithful sit on wooden pews and either read from their devotional, kneel in prayer, or silently mouth a rosary. Filtered light streams through the stained-glass windows and casts scattered splinters of gold, red, or blue sunbeams onto the sanctuary floor.

Bill slowly led me to the second pew from the front. I was a *fledgling walker* at this point in my recovery. Today was the first day in a crowd without a cane, another milestone.

The plan was to sit close enough to the altar to receive communion without being subjected to a long receiving line. I'd walk unaided back to my seat, close enough to the modesty wall to have a rail to clutch should I begin to tip. I needed something to grab other than the priest or his vestments.

The church was filling rapidly, and parishioners would soon be sitting shoulder to shoulder. A well-dressed woman settled between congregants in the row in front of me.

"Good morning," she greeted and quickly sat down.

"Morning," I responded. My eyes were drawn to a baroque-styled angel pin clasped to her shoulder. I'd never seen one quite like it before.

I bent forward and whispered, "That's a beautiful pin you're wearing."

"Thank you," she replied. A smile crossed her face. Her fingers caressed the chubby little cherub belly as she quickly turned around and bowed her head in prayer.

Before I closed my eyes, I looked intently at my hands folded in my lap, palms up. My left thumb massaged the swollen center of my right hand. I could manipulate the fingers into a straightened position, but they didn't have the strength to hold it. If I stopped rubbing, the fingers balled back into a fist.

Dear God, I know my arm is getting stronger, but I need your help to form the sign of the cross today. Two weeks ago, all that was blessed was my abdomen. It took until the final benediction to complete the motion! Last week was better. I've practiced all this week before going to sleep, but I know I'm going to still need your help. Thank you, God, for all you do. Amen.

The time of reckoning fast approached. The priest raised his hand and gracefully touched his fingertips to his forehead with reverence and said, "In the name of the Father ..."

I bent my body forward so my head was parallel to my knees. My left hand cupped my right elbow. When I pushed, it forced the arm upward and shoved the newly formed fist into my eye. I quickly regrouped and tried a second, more forceful attempt. This time, my hand jabbed my forehead with a resounding thunk. The only thing missing was me saying, "Duh."

I did whisper "Ow" under my breath.

It dawned on me that I must have looked to others like the *Thinking Man* statue and quickly dropped my arm into my lap as the priest said, "The Son ..."

I turned my hand inward and tapped my belly quickly and successfully.

Phase three was going to be the challenge. I knew my speed was one notch above neutral and my arm felt as though it were weighted with sandbags. I had to overcome the pressure of gravity.

I grabbed the wrist of my right arm with my left hand, and as the priest said, "...and the Holy Spirit," I pulled with way too much enthusiasm and slapped my left shoulder with a loud, single clap. My left hand made a straight line in front of my face, not taking into account I had a nose and uncontrollable fingers. The flailing right hand smacked the old honker hard enough to turn my face sideways (not a part of the Catholic ritual), and in a nanosecond, my right hand grabbed hold of my right shoulder, with all five fingers splayed. From the pew behind, it must have looked like Thing, (the hand on the *Addams Family*). I let go. The arm quickly dropped to the seat, pushing my elbow into the wooden back of the pew with a double knock.

I was grateful no one said, "Who's there?"

This successful attempt at making the sign of the cross must have looked like a one-man bar fight in an old-fashioned, spaghetti Western. It hadn't been a pretty sight, but man oh man I wanted to dance around the church for completing it.

As mass finished, I wore a smile of satisfaction and waited for Bill to come get me.

The woman with the angel pin slid into the pew next to me. A mixture of emotions flashed across her face.

"My friend just told me how ill you've been. You never said a word!"

Her comments poured out with no hesitation between thoughts.

"I can't believe how good you look for everything you've gone through. Are you okay?"

As she paused for breath, I responded, "I'm doing fine. Thank you for asking."

She looked at me long and hard. "You know, when you commented on my angel pin, I had an overwhelming desire to give it to you, but I didn't. I was embarrassed. I thought you'd think I was silly or something. But . . . I want you to have it. Please don't say no."

"I-I—"

"No. This is supposed to belong to you." She quickly removed it from her blouse and pinned it to my lapel.

I studied the sweet face and outreached arms of the pin.

"It's beautiful. Thank you for such a special gift. What's your name?" I asked. "I'd like to name her after you."

"Veronica. My friends call me Ronnie."

"Then that's what I'll call my new guardian angel."

———◇———

"What's the matter?" Bill asked as I pulled the seat cushions from the couch.

"I can't find my angel pin."

"You had it on when we went to church this morning."

"I know. I've worn it every day since Ronnie gave it to me last month."

Bill put his paper down. "Is it in the den?"

"No. I looked." I folded my arms as my lower lip began to pout out.

"I was just going to get some chicken wings before the football game starts. You want to come with? I'll help you look for it when we get back."

"Sure," I said and grabbed my jacket. I had to do something to get my mind off that pin.

Bill opened the car door and helped me in.

"Sweetie, look what I found!" Bill exclaimed and gently picked up the angel pin lying in the path of the car's front wheel. The pin holder was crushed. The angel's face was turned to the side and slightly tilted upward. Her arms were askew. They no longer reached outward. The left one pointed upward while the right one hung at her side.

I cradled the broken pin in my hands and looked at Bill. Tears filled my eyes. I was heartbroken. I slowly shook my head, caressed her deformed body, and quietly said, "Now she looks like me."

That night, I found a permanent home for my ravaged angel. She now sits on the corner of an ornate picture frame. Her disability allows her to only look one way, towards the face of Christ. Her good hand points as though she's introducing Him; the other hangs placidly at her side.

Ronnie's a daily reminder to me that we all have a purpose, no matter what our condition, limitation, or situation.

CHAPTER THIRTY-ONE

THE CALENDAR IS FILLING FAST

Our door was always open to company. Some people don't like visitors in their space, especially while recovering—but not us. We loved the anticipation of friends and family. To us, and all who loved us, my recovery was something to celebrate.

Lynn and her cat-from-hell (her endearment and ours) were the first to arrive. "Come on, kitty," she cooed. Lynn's nose pressed against the window of the car, her eyes scanning for fur. Fang was nowhere in sight. He'd tucked himself under the driver's seat and would make his entrance when he was good and ready.

"How long will he stay there?" I asked.

Lynn hadn't heard or seen me as I walked up behind her. "It could be hours," she replied in mid-spin. "Oh my gosh," she mouthed as she looked me up and down.

I grinned. "See? I told you I was okay."

"I'm from the *Show Me State*. I have to see it for myself. I see it ... but I don't believe it!"

"Oh, for heaven's sake," I said and hugged her. "I'm not going to break in half."

At that moment we saw a streak of fur as the wild-eyed tabby flew into the guest room from the car. He seemed grateful to no longer be in motion, but not happy. This wasn't his home. To add to the insult—he smelled D-O-G.

Molly, our three-year-old Scottie, believed everyone was her friend. It didn't matter if you stood on two feet or four, you came to play, but—she smelled C-A-T. She followed Lynn to the bedroom. The door opened. Lynn went in. The door closed. Molly was out. Her quizzical over-the-shoulder look to me seemed to say, "Can she do that?"

"Come on, girl," I called to our confused dog. She knew if she obeyed, there'd be a treat at the end of our walk.

I'd made the mistake of teaching Molly how to open doors when she was a puppy. It didn't matter if it were conventional, patio, or pocket. That little brown nose could embarrass anyone if they didn't hear the click of the privacy door before they sat down. It was just a matter of time.

It was nice to sit on the patio and visit with our friend, to catch up on all the news. Bill was the first to hear the thunderous paws of Molly. She turned the hallway corner and ran straight for the kitchen, Bill literally on her tail. She buried her front paws and face in her water bowl and then shook her head frantically. Water spilled everywhere.

"Molly, come!" Bill called.

She ran to his side, her paws wet to her chest. Water dripped from her beard and pooled on the floor. Her tongue pushed out of her mouth in long, sweeping motions.

Lynn and I ran to the bedroom fearing the worse for Fang. The door was ajar. Fang was hiding in a dresser drawer—his twitching tail the only evidence hanging from the bureau. Except his food and water dishes were empty, the trail of evidence strewn halfway down the hall.

"Molly's got grit in her mouth," Bill yelled to us.

Lynn and I laughed hysterically. "It's okay. Molly just got her first taste of kitty litter."

It was going to be a crazy few weeks. Two hours after Lynn and cat headed back to Kansas, Aunt Fran arrived. A week after that, Bill's brother, Ben. Ah, yes . . . Ben.

A white convertible with top down and radio up— way up—pulled into our driveway. Ben was visiting from Chicago. He secured the car and checked his hair in the rearview mirror before easing his way out in a classic Ferris Bueller move, sitting on the back of the driver's seat and swinging his legs over the side of the car. No need to open any door—he was too cool for that. He was in town on business with meetings scheduled at Tropicana. I wondered if he'd fess up to knowing me if anyone in his meetings made the connection between us.

The six a.m. knock on the door sounded like a police raid. "Hey! Y'all still sleeping? Let's get this party started!" he shouted through the door.

"It's going to be a full house," Bill said as he hurried to the door. He took long strides down the hallway past the family picture wall and the closed door to the guest bedroom. The dog followed closely behind, barking furiously.

"What time are the rest coming?" I called after him.

"Anytime now."

"Molly! Come here," I shouted as the dog slid between my legs, pushed the door to the guest room open with her nose, and quickly sat behind my eighty-year-old aunt, who was visiting from California. She was hoping Aunt Fran would plead mercy on her behalf; otherwise, she knew she'd be sentenced to the kitchen until everyone got here and she (the dog, not my aunt) calmed down.

Aunt Fran stood motionless, hangers scattered around her feet and across the floor. Clothing piled three feet high on one of the two twin beds, an open suitcase on the other.

"What are you doing?" I asked. "Where are you going?"

"I can't stay here."

Her face was flushed, and she was short of breath from racing between closet and dresser to suitcase.

"Why not?"

"Joanie, I'm too old. You can't expect me to share this room with Ben. I don't care if you have twin beds. I'm not that kind of woman."

I couldn't hold the guffaw any longer. "Aunt Fran, he has his own condo on the beach."

I've never seen such a look of relief. As I gave her a hug, she whispered, "Please don't tell him what a foolish old lady I am."

"I won't. Let's see if we can get this stuff hung up as fast as you got it down."

CHAPTER THIRTY-TWO

WHO'S IN CHARGE?

IT WAS A STUDY in contortion packing the car for a trip to the outlet mall with two elderly ladies (one in a wheelchair and one pushing ninety), me with my cane, a man over six feet tall, a healthy, middle-aged woman, and one teenager with an attitude and electronics attached . . . all demanding priority seating.

We looked like a clown car from a circus act as we pulled up to the curb. Bodies kept rolling out. Aunt Fran draped her purse strap around the hand rests on the back of the wheelchair and anxiously waited for Ben to transfer Bill's mom into the chair. As soon as her weight landed in the seat, they were on a roll, zipping past the stores. Aunt Fran scanned sales posters with the trained eye of a seasoned shopper. Ben went in search of the elusive parking spot as Diane and I slowly walked behind the old ladies. Pam stared at her phone, hoping someone would save her from a day of shopping with the old folks.

I was elated to be walking without my cane (left

intentionally in the car). My steps were cautious and slow, a little unsteady, especially in a crowd. If bumped, I could end up on the ground much to my chagrin and the surprise of the people nearby.

We marched into a clothing store single file, each of us focused on a different rack of clothes. We each had our own idea of what Mom would like to wear. After all, the clothes we bought today were her gift for Mother's Day.

Mom sat patiently as we paraded outfits past her and waited for her nod of approval or a thumb's down to take it back. If she nodded her head yes, the item was placed on her lap. It wasn't long before all we saw were two legs, the wheels on her chair, and a puff of snowy white hair on the crown of her head.

"Watch my purse, Joanie. I have to find a washroom," Aunt Fran announced.

"Okay," I answered. I glanced to make sure it was still hanging from the handles on the back of Mom's chair.

"I've got to find a phone," Pam mumbled and left the store. "My battery's dead."

I could see Diane walking toward Mom and me as Ben slipped through the front door as if on a mission.

"Ben and I want to check out the sunglass sale next door," she said. "We'll be right back."

"Okay," I answered hesitantly. This mass exodus left me, Mom, and the pile of clothes huddled next to the sales counter. We were on our own.

I lifted a pile of outfits from Mom's lap until I could see her face. "Are you okay in there?"

She smiled and nodded her head yes. Her beautiful blue eyes danced with delight.

"May I help you?" the saleswoman asked. She took the clothes I'd draped over a chair and hung them in a nearby dressing room.

"Yes," I replied. "We need to make a selection from these outfits."

I handed her the ones in my arms, and as I reached for the rest on Mom's lap, I froze in mid-movement. Aunt Fran's purse was no longer on the back of the chair. I looked on the floor; wrestled through the merchandise on the rack; poked around on Mom's lap and behind her back, and came up with nothing. It was gone.

Panic left a lump the size of a grapefruit in my throat.

I tapped the clerk on the shoulder. My face was flush from dread. "Excuse me. I need to find my aunt." I bent down and whispered to Mom where I was going and why.

"Where are the washrooms?" I asked. The woman gave me an all-knowing nod and a general sweep of her hand toward the front door.

The circular courtyard was a massive span of beige cobblestone with a huge fountain as the focal center point. Four manatee sculptures wearing colorful Hawaiian shirts and carrying shopping bags were positioned facing east, west, north, and south to welcome visitors from the four corners of the world. Other than the ornate fountain, everything about the terrain looked the same to me. Each shop had the same tinted glass panels trimmed in strips of dark metal. Every entrance was a double door. Even the shoppers clad in T-shirts and shorts became anonymous.

I took one giant step forward and abruptly stopped. My head was spinning from side to side.

"Dang it! I don't remember where she said the washrooms were," I muttered under my breath.

What if Aunt Fran isn't there? What if I get there and can't find my way back? What if I get lost? How will the family find me? What if they forget to look? What if they're so mad at me because the purse is missing that they don't bother to look? What if I have another stroke right here . . . right now? Nobody knows me!

I leaned against the building and tried not to gasp for air. *One step at a time*, I coaxed. *You can do this.* I forced myself to take slow, easy breaths.

There was a bench next to the southern-facing manatee straight ahead some forty feet away. That became my compass rose. I cautiously stepped forward, left, then right. My right arm still did not swing in cadence with my steps; it just hung at my side, oblivious to its role in balance.

I studied the faces of the shoppers as they passed by. *Don't they know? Can't they tell?* I felt like an imposter among the able-bodied. I wanted to shout, *I don't know where I am!*

My body began to tremble by the time I reached the bench. I made it with a mixed sense of relief and pride. I took only two lilts to the left and one to the right when my feet followed a direction all their own. I didn't realize it, but I let out an audible "Yes" as I plopped down. It startled the woman sitting at the far end of the same bench.

Out of habit, my left thumb rubbed the palm of my right hand. With my hands bound together, I pointed first at where I'd been and then where I wanted to go. Lord have mercy, I looked like I was taking aim at the mall's shoppers. I quickly placed my hand in my lap and hoped no one alerted security.

"I have to look for signs!" I exclaimed out loud. I smiled because of the profound thought I'd made. "Look for a sign!"

The stranger slid her body to the edge of our bench so only one cheek sat comfortably. Her free leg was ready to run. She casually gathered her belongings close to her side and eased the rest of her body to a standing position. With one final glance over her shoulder, she was gone.

I chuckled as a feeling of delight washed over me. The large sun bonnet my bench mate wore had obscured the tiny, inconspicuous washroom sign. I could barely keep my feet on the ground. The facility was one floppy hat and a couple of steps away. I did it. I found it by myself. It was right here!

The door to the washroom flew open. Aunt Fran walked out, still drying her hands, her purse snugly tucked under her arm.

"I thought someone stole your purse."

"No. I changed my mind. I guess you didn't hear me."

CHAPTER THIRTY-THREE

CURLS AND COWLICKS

OUR NEIGHBOR PULLED HER car into our driveway and stopped. The tinted window opened to burkah height, revealing only her eyes. They stared, unblinking, at my head.

"I have to admit," Connie said as diplomatically as possible as the window rolled open, "your hair does have a mind of its own."

I swiveled my head from side to side so she could see the full view. "I call it a bed-hair bob."

She rolled her eyes, handed me her hairstylist's well-worn card, and said, "Here. Call this number. Ask for Sheri." Then she waved out the window and sped off.

"Thank you!" I called after her and walked back to the house.

It's impossible to spend so many hours during a day in a prone position and not gain uncontrolled clusters of hair shooting out at right angles, I thought as I used my fingers to tuck the runaway curls behind my ears. Cowlicks started at the nape of my neck and ended at the crown on my left—the side I favor when I sleep.

We'd been in our new home six months when the stroke occurred. I'd not been to a beauty shop since we moved to Florida a little over nine months ago. This was long overdue.

"So, will you drive me there?" I asked.

Bill chewed and swallowed the last bite of his sandwich. "I'll drop you off, but I'm not staying." He took a swig of beer and followed it with a manly shudder at the thought of being trapped by girlie bling. "Bobby pins, rollers, and curling irons aren't my thing."

"That's fine," I replied. We both knew his favorite hardware store was a few blocks away.

He laid my cane in the back seat. "Use it," he commanded.

I obediently nodded, even though we both knew that stick wasn't leaving the car.

He turned on the windshield wipers as we pulled onto the street. Florida's weather is fickle, especially during the summer months. Most afternoons, spotty showers creep up and the skies open and pour torrents. Today was no exception. Rivers of water rushed down the roadway. Lightning pierced the ground around us with some of the strikes close enough to make us jump.

"Welcome to Florida. Lightning capital of the world," said the disc jockey on the radio.

"After that last strike," Bill responded, "I believe him."

By the time we got to the salon, the storm became a gentle patter of lingering drops. Sunlight sparkled in the puddles and steam rose from the pavement. I gazed out the car window. The smell of rain mingled with freshly mowed grass made me feel giddy. The world seemed more beautiful and magical than I remembered.

"I'll be back in an hour," Bill said as I kissed him good-bye.

"I'll be waiting." I caught sight of the cane in the back seat but didn't say a word. I watched as the car rounded the corner onto Manatee Avenue and drove out of sight.

The hedge of blooming ixora partially hid the ramp/stairs leading to the salon's side entry. I felt a tinge of fear squelching my excitement.

The people on the other side of that door are strangers. What if I start to cry? What if I cry ugly!? No one will understand.

That thought alone was enough to make tears appear. I blinked hard and gulped twice.

What if I can't find the right words to describe the cut I want? What if Bill's late picking me up? I don't know for sure where he went.

The salon, located on the first floor of the turn-of-the-century Tudor home, had its entrance off the side yard near the back of the house. It reminded me of the door we used at Grandma's, the one that welcomed friends and family. This one had that same feeling of *come on in and set a spell.*

The six panes of glass in the brightly colored, yellow door were covered with stark white, open-laced curtains—both drawn back from the middle with a sash.

"Bye, Sheri! We'll see you next month," the young mother with three kids in tow shouted over her shoulder. I heard a tinkle of bells as she closed the door behind her. The brood scurried towards the waiting SUV. The mom's fingers flipped the long, gently curling locks Sheri had just trimmed. Wow . . . she looked gorgeous.

A muffled din of conversations from the other side of the door sounded cheerful enough before the door closed.

I took a deep breath as my internal cheerleader prodded, "You can do this."

I placed my hand on the round doorknob and confidently turned it. My hand twisted one hundred eighty degrees. The knob stayed in place. I began to realize my biggest *what-if* question should have been—*What if I can't get the darn door open?*

I stood helplessly, under the dripline of the gutter above the doorway, and watched people in the salon go about their business. A steady cadence of raindrops trickled from the leaves gorged in the gutter's channel. Rogue drops landed on top of my bangs, trailed down my nose, and with a steady drip, bounced to the ground.

I gripped the handle with my right hand, my left firmly on top. This time, standing sideways, I used my full body weight and twisted the knob forward. My right leg rose off the ground, swinging freely from the knee.

My body lurched fore and aft. The movements looked like those of a figurine on a seventeenth-century German chime clock. The knob held its position through it all as though it had been polished with butter. I prayed no one inside saw this spectacle through the door's window.

I briefly thought about tapping one of the panes in the hopes someone would hear. But with the water dripping from my nose, my hair flying in all directions, and a slanted mouth that changed from a smile to a frown quicker than a blinking neon sign, it made me decide against it. I stood, peering in the window, looking like a waif from one of Dickens's novels: "Please, someone, won't you let me in?"

As I lifted the tail on my blouse from within my pants like a magician pulling silk scarves from his sleeve, a woman came running up the steps behind me.

"Excuse me," she said.

With pure joy, I let her pass. She opened the door and I caught the edge of it with my left hand and followed her in.

I brushed at my top as though raindrops were still caught in my clothes. My plan to use the cloth of my blouse to gain traction on the door knob was no longer necessary.

"Boy, that's some storm," I said to the receptionist and shoved my blouse back into place. She glanced out the window and then looked at me with a "Huh?" expression. The sun was shining brightly.

I sighed.

"I'm here to see Sheri."

She nodded her head toward the end of the room. Her eyes stayed focused on the twenty shades of pink nail color sitting on the counter before her.

A pretty woman ... thirtyish, with large doe eyes and shimmering, dark brown hair cascading to her waist walked towards me. She listened carefully as I described the style I wanted.

"I need to explain something before we begin," I slurred and hesitated. "Sometimes I have difficulty controlling my tears and laughter. It's called lability."

"I never heard of it."

"I recently had a stroke. Lability is a side effect that comes from it. Sometimes it can be funny. Sometimes, it's just downright embarrassing. I never know when it will happen.

"Why would a stroke cause that?" she asked.

"I don't know the medical explanation. The best way I can describe it to you is this way: If you've ever watched a scary horror movie and someone startles you to the point your popcorn flies through the air and you laugh, then cry, and laugh again. It's like that ... only over and over. Having a stroke is terrifying. If you survive it, you'll go through this laughing and crying phase. They say it will gradually end, but in the meantime ..."
I just raised my hands to hide my face and shook my head.

She fluffed the black, plastic cape and draped it over my shoulders.

"That's okay, sweetie. I'll only take it personally if you cry after I finish your cut."

I began to laugh.

CHAPTER THIRTY-FOUR

INDEPENDENCE DAY

My body was recovering at warp speed: eyesight normal, speech almost lucid. Physically, no one could tell I endured a stroke, except for the swelling and nerve damage in my right hand. Doctors said in time that should return, as well.

Bill was standing in the driveway, holding onto the handlebar of my bike. "You said you wanted to ride again. I think you're ready."

My heart skipped a beat in anticipation.

"Take it slow. Get your balance," Bill coached. He ran alongside, his hand on the underside of the bike's seat.

I could feel myself pulling away from his grip as my feet gained momentum on the pedals.

"Don't go too far!" he shouted. He stood in the middle of the street with a grin as wide as the road.

I felt free. No, normal. I felt normal.

I rode to the end of the block and back, which meant to our driveway in the middle of the block. Bill and my sister-in-law jumped in a circle, high-fiving each other and yelling. You'd think I'd won the Tour de France.

Bill grabbed me and swung me around. "I'm so proud of you!" He held my shoulders and looked me square in the eyes. "You know what I'm going to say, don't you?"

I nodded. "If I can ride a bike, I can drive a car."

"You've been driving to the store and back with me in my car, and you've done just fine. It's time you venture out on your own."

I hadn't sat in my car since the stroke. I wasn't sure I wanted to.

"Why don't you visit Mom?" he suggested. "She'd love it."

"You want me to go to St. Petersburg?"

"Why not?"

"That's thirty miles away!"

A huge picture of a man and a woman dressed in WWII vintage clothing rested on an easel outside the activity center's doorway a few feet from mom's room. "Enjoy the Good Old Days—Today!" read the poster. The large crowd, sitting in a semicircle, listened to the couple sing songs from the forties. Some of the patrons were holding hands, others tapped their toes or hummed along. The man played the piano while the woman flirted with the audience in between tunes.

I lightly rapped on Mom's closed door. Her back was

turned. She was watching television, and the sound was blaring.

"Hi, Mom!" I yelled. "What're you doing in here? The party's out there." I gave her a kiss.

She looked at me in dismay and then glanced at the door. Her eyes and facial expressions had become her voice since a stroke left her unable to speak six years ago.

"Bill?" She nodded her head.

"He's at home."

A look of puzzlement crossed her face.

"I drove myself. He said I could do it. He was right." She looked at me in disbelief.

"See what your prayers have done?"

She nodded her head vigorously. A smile lit up her face.

"Why are we sitting in here, Ma? The party's down the hall. They're starting to serve strawberry shortcake."

She waved her hand with an air of disdain. She hated to mix and mingle. She was deaf, and being in crowd chatter was difficult at best. However, this time, the shortcake won her over. Mom's eyes widened with glee as she reached for a fork. I was right behind her.

We had a wonderful visit, talking about nothing in particular and everything family. There's something about being with a parent, even one who's aging, that brings the world into balance and makes you feel whole.

The air was warm, but the breeze was picking up on the ride home. Large thunder clouds formed in the east. Another hour and we'd have the expected afternoon summer shower. I'd be home before then.

I loved the view across Tampa Bay from the one-hundred-eighty-foot-high Sunshine Skyway Bridge. The brilliant colors of the windsurfers' sails zipping across the turquoise/teal-blue gulf waters and the occasional breech of bottlenose dolphins left me spellbound. These young men and women had such a zest and daring for life. Even when they fell, they'd get back up and do it again.

The view made me realize life is always going to be filled with challenges, but it was also brilliantly beauti-ful. The choice I needed to make for myself was—Am I going to be a spectator or a player? It was up to me, and either one was acceptable, but which would keep me productive and make me happy? For me that choice was clear.

As I drove down I-75, I thought about how grateful I was for all I had, especially an amazing husband who was making his infamous homemade spaghetti sauce for dinner tonight. It doesn't get much better than that.

—⁂—

I'd become comfortable enough with driving in the past few weeks that I didn't give it a thought anymore.

The cuckoo clock chimed ten. "I'll be home around

four o'clock," I shouted to Bill, who was flipping channels in the other room.

I counted the film, cleaned and checked the lenses in my camera bag, and squirrelled a pair of sunglasses into a side pocket. "I'm really looking forward to visiting Selby Gardens today. I've heard such good things about it."

"Have a great time," Bill said. He loaded the gear and tripod into the trunk of the car, stepped back, and surveyed the mountain of gadgets. "Are you sure you can handle all this?"

"No," I said with a shrug. I looked at the pile of equipment that could bring a pack animal to its knees. "I guess I'll figure out what I need when I get there and leave the rest in the trunk."

Bill sensed the apprehension in my voice.

"You're going to do just fine. Take your time. If you tire, sit and rest. Most of all, enjoy the day."

I always felt better with his arms around me as they were now. It made me feel sure of myself and what I could accomplish.

"Thank you, honey," I said and pulled my arms around his middle with a pat to the belly.

"Sounds ripe to me."

"Me, too," he said and sucked it in until his face turned red.

"Linda told me she packed a picnic basket for our girl's day out. Wine for her, diet soda for me," I snickered. "Several rooty-tooty cheeses, smoked sausages, fresh fruit, and an assortment of crackers."

"Stop! You're making me hungry." He held his stomach.

"I don't feel any sympathy for you. You've got chicken wings." I pointed at the plate in his hand.

He took a big bite and licked his lips. "You say hello to Dave; I'll say hello to this." His mouth closed around another wing. Sauce dribbled down his chin.

"I will." I blew him a kiss. He waved, wing in hand.

Linda and I discovered we both had a passion for photography while I was in the rehab facility, and she was helping me regain my voice. The first two photo safaris we took were to the beach. She drove. This time, I was driving. It was a thirty-minute ride to her house. She lived a short, ten-minutes from the garden and a block from Sarasota Bay. I'm sure thoughts of my wheelchair maneuvering at the rehab center crossed her mind as she waited for her ride. I know it did mine.

The weather was ideal for picture taking. Cotton ball clouds billowed across the vibrant blue sky. It rained last night. Everything looked fresh in the early morning sunlight. Tiny sprouts of new growth added another dimension of color to the palette, perfect for photography.

I pulled onto the white, crushed-shell driveway and walked through the open-air portico of the rambling, Spanish-style home. I could see someone coming to the door.

"Hey, y'all!" I greeted in the southern accent I'd been practicing.

After a long pause and lengthy stare, I realized it wasn't the wisest greeting to use with a language therapist.

"Hello," she said hesitantly, still gawking.

"Are you ready to go?" I asked.

"You bet." She grabbed her belongings piled next to the front door.

"Do you need some help?" I reached for the picnic basket.

"No, no. I've got it."

Dave came lumbering up the hallway from the kitchen, his hands full of snacks. He was ready for the game. When he saw Linda struggling with the bags, he came running to help.

She kissed him as though it were their last good-bye. I wondered if she regretted agreeing to ride with a stroke survivor driving. I think I may have.

"We won't be late," she told her husband. Her fingertips lingered on his. "It should be a fun day."

Her mouth may have said *fun* but her eyes pleaded "Help me!"

"Bill says hi, Dave." He's doing the same thing you are, watching the game." I unlocked the car door.

"Hi back!" he yelled. It was hard to hear him over the sound of crushing shells as the car rolled out of the drive.

"I'm looking forward to visiting Selby Gardens," I said. A wash of excitement swept over me. "I've never been before."

"Oh! I've been a member of their garden club for years. Today's the last day of the orchid show. You're going to see thousands of varieties, and that's no exaggeration. I didn't want you or me to miss this event."

"How large is the campus?"

"It's fifty-one acres of botanical beauty on the bay near the heart of downtown Sarasota." She groaned. "I sound like an ad!"

"Naw. Just . . . Yeah, you do," I laughed.

"I can't help it. Some of the specimens grown there are one of a kind. The garden is small, compared to others across our nation, but it's absolutely a hidden treasure on the Suncoast.

I'm also looking forward to seeing the newly renovated reception hall," she added. "We're thinking of renting the space for our daughter's wedding."

"You seem to know a lot about the grounds."

"Uh-huh."

I saw her eyes glue to an approaching car. Linda was visibly nervous about riding with me driving, although she wasn't about to say so.

Her gestures were over exaggerated and calculated as she fastened her seat belt. Her feet rested firmly on the invisible brake used when teaching teens to drive the family car. Her right hand casually clenched the shoulder harness, and she nestled her back firmly into the seat. Every muscle in her body was rigid.

Traffic was light and steady as we made our way toward Tamiami Trail.

"So," she began. Her voice cracked like a prepubescent teenage boy talking to the hottest girl in school. She cleared her throat and started, again. "So, how long have you been driving?"

A wry smile began to form. Darn that thalamus ... I couldn't hold back. I casually replied, "Since I was seventeen."

PART SEVEN

LESSONS LEARNED

CHAPTER THIRTY-FIVE

LIVING AS A STROKE SURVIVOR

I WAS VERY TIRED today. I don't do well when I'm tired. My hand began to swell and ache; my speech slurred more than usual, and my balance was slightly off. I knew these symptoms wouldn't last. At least, I hoped they won't.

On good days when I feel wonderful, I like to say I'm new and improved. When those precious days appear, I work too hard, play too hard, shop too long, and visit too late. I act normal and the following day, I pay. That's what I did yesterday. So today? I pay.

I curse myself for not having the common sense of a lima bean to pace myself. I take my vitals and swear the end is imminent, even though everything appears fine. I have to accept the results on fact and faith, even though I doubt them both.

I needed to leave soon. My peer training classes with the local hospital therapy department were now over.

Today, the Stroke Support Peer Visitor Group met with patients for the first time.

"You look nice," Bill said, admiring what he saw.

"Thank you," I replied.

"Are you excited?"

"Yeah, but I don't know what to expect. I have a truckload of knowledge crammed into my brain, but I'm not sure I'll say what they need to hear."

"It's going to be different with each person, you know."

"That's what Shawna told me, too. She said to let the patient lead the conversation—I can do that."

I looked at the watch I wore (for decoration) and gasped. "Oh my gosh! I've got to go."

A calendar still means nothing to me. However, when an event looms, it consumes my thoughts, but that's all it does. I have no concept of planning for it or implementing it. It just converts to a stationary, ever-present thought. I've been told the more involved I become with life, the more important time will be. Eventually, as I compartmentalize time into fifteen-minute increments, it's supposed to reconnect in my mind.

When I told Bill this theory, he just gave me *that* look and said, "We'll see, honey. For you, time's a wire that's always been crimped."

As I drove to the medical complex, I thought about what Shawna told us the last day of training: "The success of healing depends not only on the ability and willingness of the patient to respond, but the willingness of the medical staff, family, and friends to help set and achieve goals."

We received our final pep talk this morning in the conference room.

"The reason we developed the Stroke Support Peer Visitor Program is to offer courage, knowledge, and hope to the stroke survivor who's just beginning this uncharted journey. We believe if the patient sees and talks to someone who's endured a stroke, already faced rehab, and returned to an active, albeit altered, lifestyle, it will encourage the recovering patient to get back to living."

I thought about the people I'd meet today and prayed.

"Just remember, each person is different," Shawna said before we headed to our assigned floor. "Depending on where the brain attack occurred, the symptoms will be unique. Their need for encouragement, comfort, and caution will be as individual as they are. By the way, if they believe they can accomplish something outside their abilities, encourage them to talk it over with their family and medical team, always stress safety first, and don't forget to fill out the visitor/patient report."

～⁓～

I met Alana, a hospital volunteer friend of mine, in the coffee shop after we made our rounds. She was a cheerful and spry eighty year old who walked with a slight limp (residual from a stroke three years ago). She carried an ornate cane, one decorated with sequins and the occasional Cheerio—one that her grandchildren decorated as a birthday surprise last week. When I saw her from behind, that little lilt reminded me of a Broadway dancer practicing a show tune that played only in her head.

"So, how'd it go?" she asked.

I set my tray on the table. "I can't believe how open and friendly everyone was."

"You can't ask for a better response than that," she replied.

I stirred my bowl of vegetable soup to cool it down, opened a packet of crackers, and began to butter. "Let me ask you something that someone asked me this morning."

"Sure. Go ahead," she replied. She rested her elbows on the table and leaned forward.

"If someone asked you to tell them in one word what lesson you learned from having a stroke, what would you say?"

She thought for a moment before responding, "Gratitude."

"Me too." I smiled. "In fact, that's what I told her."

"I live with a new set of priorities," Alana said with conviction. "I appreciate the important things in life: God, family, friends—all the things that aren't things."

I nodded in agreement.

"I tell people," Alana said, wagging her finger, "don't involve me in your pettiness or drama. That's the heartbeat for misery, and I don't live there," she tapped her finger on the table, "anymore!"

I took a sip of water. "Since my stroke, and for the

first time in my life, I've been open to unconditional love. People see me for who and what I am. They love me anyway."

"Go figure," Alana interrupted. She smiled and patted my hand.

"I know." I shrugged my shoulders and shook my head. "The more surprising thing is, I saw myself as they did. No judgement. No anger."

We placed our trays on the counter and walked to our cars.

"I'm not the same as I was before the stroke," I added. "Before, it never crossed my mind that my body would betray me."

"Not in the infancy of middle age," Alana added. "You were so young when it happened to you. But then it can happen at any age, even children."

"True. But for people of vintage age, like us, did you ever feel like mortality is ticking a countdown?"

"Time. Is. Running. Out!" Alana chided robotically.

"No. I'm serious," I said. "I feel I need to complete my life's mission, whatever it is and wherever it takes me, before my journey is over and this body makes its final exit."

"Yep." Alana nodded. "A handshake with death sets your priorities straight, that's for sure."

CHAPTER THIRTY-SIX

EVERY BODY'S DIFFERENT

BILL AND I LIVE in a boating community in Florida. I love touring the new home models and would probably use any excuse to visit them, but today I was on a mission. Bill sent me to measure the length from the table top to the chandelier hanging over the dining room table in the model we chose. I gladly volunteered.

The life-sized pictures hanging in the showroom were magnificent representations of warm-weather living. Sleek boats, sandy beaches, blazing red sunsets, and exotic birds drew potential home owners closer to the door leading to the models. We know these scenes. We know what happens next. The display reeled us in last year.

"If you lived here, you'd be home by now" read the stylized sign hanging above the doorway. It was etched on a piece of seasoned driftwood. I smiled, knowing a short, three-block drive to the east led to our front door.

This was our dream, a dream that became reality six months before the stroke. It's a dream we were beginning to enjoy nearly a year later. Our lifestyle was beginning to return to normal. I was home—free from institutional living and therapy, grateful for every new day and all that it offered.

A flash of white passed the sales office's windows and parked in the handicapped space closest to the door. I thought for a moment it was my friend's car, but instead, an older couple walked into the design center, retirees from New York.

"You work here?" Dominic asked.

"No. I live here. I'm just waiting for someone."

"You live here, huh? You like it?"

"We love it."

"We're looking for a place in the sun. I can't take the cold weather up north anymore. Not since my stroke."

"You had a stroke?" I was shocked!

His posture was good, no telltale droop to his face. Speech seemed perfect. Arms and legs moved in sync.

"You don't show any of the signs. You look wonderful." Before I could stop myself I blurted out, "I had one, too."

He grabbed my hand and shook it hard. I felt like I was in the clutch of a bear.

"How long ago for you?" he asked.

"Nearly a year."

"Nine years for me," he responded. His face clouded with gloom.

He bent his head toward my ear. "We live on disability," he replied softly.

You could tell for someone who'd lived through the Great Depression, being dependent was a bitter pill, indeed.

"We're looking to move someplace where it's not as expensive." His searching eyes looked at me long and hard. "Someplace warm."

"You're in the right state," I answered cheerfully.

His gaze focused on my lips. "Your speech, was it affected?"

"Yeah. Yeah it was."

"Any paralysis?"

"Whole right side—couldn't talk, couldn't walk, couldn't stand, couldn't see straight."

"But . . . you look fine," he said in complete bafflement. "Tell her, Gladys, she looks fine!"

"You look fine, dear."

I gave them both a hug. "You look fine, too, Dominic."

I felt a sorrow within him. His body may have healed, but the trauma of the event lived on in his memories—a never-ending loop of surrender for what he had and believed would never have again. He'd placed himself within the confining walls of *can't* instead of surrounding himself with the anticipation of *can try*. It's no wonder he wore a mantle of hopelessness.

As a stroke survivor, I learned quickly that we have no control over the stroke itself, or whether we live or die. Only our attitude for facing the crisis can be adjusted. I had to come to terms with Dr. Elisabeth Kübler

Ross's stages of grief (more than once, sometimes) before I could begin to heal. As difficult as it was, it was necessary to face the denial and shock of the event; the guilt of doing better when others were not; the anger and bargaining because I was forever altered and unsure of the future; and the depression from knowing others now saw me as someone who was disabled. Finally, I found a modicum of peace and acceptance. There were many nights of reflection and depression, knowing I may never be the same again. Fighting to recover from a stroke is a struggle like no other, yet it's one worth battling.

I'm grateful to know, after my ordeal, there's nothing to fear from death. A sense of peace and destiny were all encompassing at the height of the event. Any transgressions I had on my soul were unimportant at that moment. I realized God forgives us all, no matter what, if we're truly sorry. We are the ones who struggle with forgiving others and ourselves.

If I'd spent more time with Dominic and Gladys, I wondered if I would have said that. Irony curled the left side of my lip when I realized our most brilliant conversations take place after the other person is gone. Well, what I thought was in my heart, and maybe, someday, I'd be able to share it with someone else, for what it's worth.

I believe as long as we have breath, we have hope, and as long as we are alive, no matter what our circumstances, we may live with peace and joy. That's our choice.

Never give up trying. Even if we never regain what we've lost, we may find other talents that have been hidden until now. All our lives we redefine ourselves as we mature. Why stop now?

Keep on living!

CHAPTER THIRTY-SEVEN

DON'T GIVE UP

"These turned out really nice," Shawna said as she handed me a stack of cards printed on bright yellow paper.

I'd approached her a few weeks prior with an idea for the patients who were not in their rooms when we stopped to visit.

"Why not leave them a note, one that would speak directly to them—a note with messages written from one survivor to another?"

"This was a great idea. Thank you," she said. "You're the first to use them."

"Thank you. And you're welcome," I responded. "They did turn out nice," I said as I placed the cards into my briefcase.

I checked the roster and headed for the elevator.

In the very first room, I could see two pairs of feet jutting out from the visitor's chairs next to the patient's bed but no patient in sight.

I crossed myself and said a quick prayer before entering.

"Good morning." I quickly scanned the room and checked the roster. "Is this Miss Ivy's room?"

"Yes," the older man nodded.

"Are you Miss Ivy's family?"

The middle-aged woman replied, "I'm her daughter. This is her husband."

"I take it she's somewhere in the building having tests done."

They glanced at each other as they nodded.

"Let me introduce myself, and if you have any questions, please feel free to ask." I searched my briefcase for a copy of the card.

"I found myself in a similar situation about a year ago."

"Was it your spouse?"

"No. It was me. I was the patient."

Surprise registered on their faces.

"Let me tell you why I'm here," I said and closed the door.

THE END

A PERSONAL NOTE

I HOPE YOU ENJOYED reading *Trapped Within* and that it gave you some insight, or peace, or motivation to keep living life to the fullest—even if it's necessary to safely readjust the ways you approach life.

The following are words of encouragement that helped motivate and reassure me during my recovery. I hope you'll find something here to inspire or comfort you, or someone you love.

- Be Good to Yourself—Wash Away Negative Thoughts.

- Exercise Patience and Perseverance.

- You Are *Not* a Victim. YOU ARE A SURVIVOR.

- Set Goals—Reach for Them—Adjust When You Must.

- Take All the Time You Need. Just Don't Quit!

- You May Not Be the Same—You May Be Better!

- Love Yourself—Forgive Yourself, Forgive Others—Let It Go.

- Kindness and Laughter Are the Best Elixirs for Healing.

- It Does Get Better.
  – Written by: Jo Ann V. Glim

OTHER BOOKS
BY JO ANN GLIM

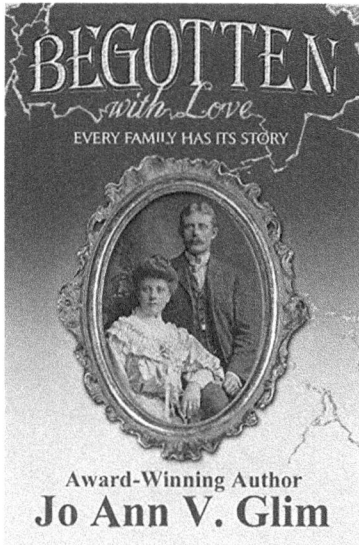

Award-Winning Author
Jo Ann V. Glim

IF YOU ENJOY BIOG-RAPHIES, you may want to read *Begotten with Love: Every Family Has Its Story,* a Florida Writers Association Royal Palm Literary Award first-place winner for biography.

Imagine receiving a Bible from the 1800s which contained a portion of your family's genealogy and then hearing this cryptic message from your aunt, "By the way, your maiden name is not Elliott." This was the beginning of a thirty year search for identity and truth. One hundred fifty years of American history and five generations of family revealed a vision of honor and webs of deceit, but when a stranger called— a sixty-five-year-old mystery was finally exposed.

TESTIMONIALS

"THIS IS DEFINITELY A testament to hope, love, and forgiveness, and a wonderfully crafted tale that will keep your attention from beginning to end."   – SHARON M.

"IT READS LIKE FICTION, but it's not!"   – BOB M.

**More on Amazon.com and
www.Goodreads.com/JoAnnGlim**

SPREAD THE WORD

IF YOU ENJOYED *TRAPPED Within*, the best way to let others know is to leave a review on Amazon (five stars means you loved it). If you'd like to be kept up to date about book signings, contests, and events, follow or like us on Facebook, and/or join our email list to find out what we're planning next. We will be respectful of your time and email space. No Spam.

We know your reading time is limited, and if you're like the rest of us, the books you want to read are stacked to the ceiling. I am humbled and happy you chose *Trapped Within*. Thank you.

BOOK CLUBS / TEACHERS / MEDICAL PROFESSIONALS

INTERESTED IN BULK / wholesale purchases for your group or workshop? Email a request to JoAnnGlim. author@gmail.com.

BOOK CLUB DISCUSSION QUESTIONS are available now

TEACHER'S GUIDE AVAILABLE SOON.

KEEP IN TOUCH

IF YOU KNOW SOMEONE who may benefit from this book, please, let them know it's available on-line through all major book sellers.

WOULD YOU LIKE TO CONTACT ME? HERE'S HOW:

FACEBOOK / TWITTER / YouTube / or our website, www.JOANNGLIM.COM

JOANNGLIM.AUTHOR@GMAIL.COM
PO BOX 174, BRADENTON, FL 34206

YOUR PURCHASE HELPS OTHERS
IN NEED

I BELIEVE IN GIVING BACK. A portion of the proceeds from our sales support charities such as the Academic Crossroads Memorial Endowment Scholarship (ACME) fund. This fund assists students whose educational opportunities are in jeopardy due to the death of a sibling or parent. For more information, visit my website: www.JoAnnGlim.com/Scholarship.

IF YOU THINK YOU'RE HAVING
A STROKE DO NOT IGNORE
THE WARNING SIGNS
GET HELP IMMEDIATELY!
9-1-1

www.ingramcontent.com/pod-product-compliance
Lightning Source LLC
Chambersburg PA
CBHW020250030426
42336CB00010B/706